D0890084

Federal Regulation of Methadone Treatment

WITHDRAWN

Richard A. Rettig and Adam Yarmolinsky, *Editors*

Committee on Federal Regulation of Methadone Treatment

Division of Biobehavioral Sciences and Mental Disorders

INSTITUTE OF MEDICINE

NATIONAL ACADEMY PRESS
Washington, D.C. 1995

NATIONAL ACADEMY PRESS • 2101 Constitution Avenue, N.W. • Washington, DC 20418

NOTICE: The project that is the subject of this report was approved by the governing board of the National Research Council, whose members are drawn from the councils of the National Academy of Sciences, the National Academy of Engineering, and the Institute of Medicine. The members of the committee responsible for the report were chosen for their special competencies and with regard to appropriate balance.

This report has been reviewed by a group other than the authors according to procedures approved by a report review committee consisting of members of the National Academy of Sciences, the National Academy of Engineering, and the Institute of Medicine.

The Institute of Medicine was chartered in 1970 by the National Academy of Sciences to enlist distinguished members of the appropriate professions in the examination of policy matters pertaining to the health of the public. In this the Institute acts under both the Academy's 1863 congressional charter responsibility to be an advisor to the federal government and its own initiative in identifying issues of medical care, research, and education.

Support for this project was provided by the U.S. Public Health Service pursuant to Contract No. 282-92-0079.

Library of Congress Catalog Card No. 94-74890
International Standard Book No. 0-309-05240-8

Additional copies of the report are available from:

National Academy Press
2101 Constitution Avenue, N.W.
P.O. Box 285
Washington, DC 20055

Call 800-624-6242 or 202-334-3313 (in the Washington Metropolitan Area).

B520

The serpent has been a symbol of long life, healing, and knowledge among almost all cultures and religions since the beginning of recorded history. The image adopted as a logotype by the Institute of Medicine is based on a relief carving from ancient Greece, now held at the Staatlichemuseen in Berlin.

COMMITTEE ON THE FEDERAL REGULATION OF METHADONE TREATMENT

ADAM YARMOLINSKY *(Chairman)*, Regents Professor of Public Policy in the University of Maryland System, University of Maryland, Baltimore County, Baltimore, Maryland

M. DOUGLAS ANGLIN, Director, Drug Abuse Research Center, UCLA Neuropsychiatric Institute, Los Angeles, California

JOHN C. BALL, Senior Scientist, Center for Studies on Addiction, University of Pennsylvania, School of Medicine, Philadelphia, Pennsylvania

JANICE F. KAUFFMAN, Director, Substance Abuse Treatment Services, North Charles, Inc., Harvard Medical School, Department of Psychiatry, The Cambridge Hospital, Somerville, Massachusetts

MARY JEANNE KREEK, Professor and Head of Laboratory, Laboratory on the Biology of Addictive Diseases, The Rockefeller University, New York, New York

A. THOMAS MCLELLAN, Research Professor of Psychiatry, Center for Studies on Addiction, University of Pennsylvania, School of Medicine, Philadelphia, Pennsylvania

J. THOMAS PAYTE, Founder and Medical Director, Drug Dependence Associates, San Antonio, Texas

MICHAEL L. PRENDERGAST, Drug Abuse Research Center, UCLA Neuropsychiatric Institute, Los Angeles, California

PETER REUTER, School of Public Affairs, University of Maryland, College Park, Maryland

LEE N. ROBINS, Professor of Social Science in Psychiatry, University Professor of Social Science, Department of Psychiatry, Washington University, School of Medicine, St. Louis, Missouri

RICHARD J. RUSSO, Consultant, Substance Abuse Policy, West Trenton, New Jersey

MARGUERITE T. SAUNDERS, Commissioner, Office of Alcoholism and Substance Abuse Services, State of New York, Albany, New York

LEE SECHREST, Professor, Department of Psychology, University of Arizona, Tucson, Arizona

EDWARD C. SENAY, Professor of Psychiatry, University of Chicago, Chicago, Illinois

LISA MOJER-TORRES, Attorney, Jersey City, New Jersey

WILLIAM W. VODRA, Senior Partner, Arnold & Porter, Washington, D.C.

JERRY V. WILSON, Senior Vice President, Crime Control Research Corporation, Washington, D.C.

iii

Acknowledgments

This report results from the deliberations of the Institute of Medicine Committee on Federal Regulation of Methadone Treatment and its conclusions and recommendations reflect the judgments of the committee. Support for this study was provided by the U.S. Public Health Service (Contract No. 282-92-0079).

The actual preparation of the report under the direction of the committee has been accomplished by the collective efforts of committee members, staff, and other contributors. The committee wishes to acknowledge its gratitude for these various contributions.

Thanks for assistance in the preparation of this report, the provision of information, and the checking of facts are due to many people and organizations. The New York State Office of Alcoholism and Substance Abuse Services, headed by Marguerite Saunders, a member of the committee, deserves special thanks. In particular, the following individuals provided much assistance: Addi Corradi, Vincent Fenlon, William Lachanski, John Perez, Anthony Scro, and Frank Tardalo.

The New York State Committee of Methadone Program Administrators prepared an analysis of federal regulations at the request of the Institute of Medicine. Thanks go especially to Martin Livenstein and Frank McGurk, and to their colleagues, for a document that was highly informative and very useful to the committee in the early stages of its work.   Visits to methadone clinics were made in a number of cities. Clinic visits in New York City were facilitated by Sy Dempsky and Richard Marx at Mt. Sinai Hospital Narcotic and Rehabilitation Center, Elizabeth Khuri, the Adolescent Development Program, New York Hospital and Cornell Medical College. A tour of the Rockefeller University laboratories of Mary Jeanne Kreek was arranged by Janel Maki. At Beth Israel Hospital, we met with Robert Newman, Nina Peyser, Stuart Nichols, Marie Marciano, and Donald DesJarlais, and were shown a treatment program by Lolita Silva. Massachusetts methadone program directors who met with the study director included Vincent Tobin, Edward Bloniari, Matthew Davis, Tim Schuettje, Harvey Kauffman, Norma Reppucci, Brian Foss, and Pat Rushton. Karst Besteman, director of the Substance Abuse Center, Institute for Behavior Resources, Inc., Washington, D.C., provided valuable historical information as well as a tour of two facilities. Jeffrey A. Hoffman, of Adapt, Inc., and Koba Associates, Inc., Washington, D.C., also arranged a facility tour and shared with the study the benefits of his research. In Baltimore, we visited Man Alive, courtesy of its long-time director, Richard Lane, who is now deceased. At the Sinai Hospital Drug Dependence Program in Baltimore, Franklin T. Evans hosted our visit.

Robert W. Schuster, former Director of the National Institute on Drug Abuse (NIDA), under whom this study originated, provided counsel early in the study. The oversight committee of the Department of Health and Human Services for this study included Lorraine Fishback, Office of the Assistant Secretary of Health, Nicholas Reuter, Food and Drug Administration (FDA); Dorynne Czechowicz, Steve Molinari, and James Cooper of NIDA, and Robert Lubran, Center for Substance Abuse Treatment, Substance Abuse and Mental Health Services Administration (SAMHSA). At NIDA, we also received help from Bennett Fletcher, Charles Grudzinskas, and Frank Vocci. At SAMHSA, Sue Becker, Jerome Jaffe, Herman Diesenhaus, and Mady Chalk were helpful to the study. Additional help was provided by the following individuals at the FDA: Stuart Nightingale, Curtis Wright, Betty Jones, Ellsworth Dory, and Ross Laderman.

A special note of thanks goes to David E. Joranson, associate director for Policy Studies, Pain Research Group, University of Wisconsin-Madison, for providing his own comments and stimulating communications from others to the committee regarding the effects of the methadone regulations on the management of pain.

At the Drug Enforcement Administration, Thomas Gitchel, Ann Carter, Frank Sapienza, and Howard McLain were helpful at various times during the study. At the Office of National Drug Control Policy (ONDCP), John Gregorich and Sam Schildhaus were helpful, as was Lee Brown, director of ONDCP. Peter Edelman, counsel to the Secretary of Health and Human Services, met with the chairman and study director midway in the study and provided useful guidance on the departmental perspective on drug policy.

Regarding the actual writing of the report, the first draft of chapter 1 was prepared by Richard Rettig and then reviewed extensively by the entire committee. Chapter 2 was written by Mary Jeanne Kreek. Sally Satel assisted on an early draft and Constance Pechura also provided helpful assistance. Chapter 3 was written by Lee Robins and Douglas Anglin. Robins conducted special analyses of the Epidemiologic Catchment Area study data for this chapter. Anglin received assistance in analyzing drug use forecasting data from Vincent Fenlon in the New York State Office of Alcoholism and Substance Abuse Services, Susan Nisenbaum in the California Department of Alcohol and Drug Programs, and Talbert Cottey, at the National Institute of Justice, and for data analysis from Jessie Hsieh and Mel Widawski, at the University of

California, Los Angeles Drug Abuse Research Center.

Chapter 4 was written by Michael Prendergast, who was assisted by Dana Baldwin. Chapter 5 was written by Richard Rettig, who benefited from extensive documentation provided by Steve Molinari and James Cooper of NIDA, and from presentations to the committee by Peter Hutt, Jerome Jaffe, and Stewart Nightingale. Chapter 6 was written by Miriam Davis, consultant to the committee. She wishes to acknowledge the assistance of Daniel Melnick and Robert Lubran, SAMHSA; Elsworth Dory, FDA; Ralph Swindle, Veterans Affairs Medical Center, Palo Alto, Department of Veterans Affairs; Henrick Harwood and Douglas Fountain, Lewin-VHI, Inc.; Thomas D'Aunno, University of Michigan;, Helen Levine Batten, Brandeis University; William Butynski, National Association of State Alcohol and Drug Abuse Directors; Mark Parrino, American Methadone Treatment Association; Addie Corradi, New York State Office of Alcoholism and Substance Abuse Services; Joy Jarfors, California Department of Alcohol and Drug Programs; Phil Emenheiser, Florida Department of Health and Rehabilitative Services; Richard Weisskopf, Illinois Department of Alcoholism and Substance Abuse; and Barbara Espey, Massachusetts Department of Public Health. Chapter 7 was written by Janice Kauffman, Thomas Payte, and Thomas McLellan. Chapter 8 was written by Richard Rettig.

Thelma Cox, with patience, good humor, and grace, supported the project throughout its duration and prepared the many drafts and the camera-ready copy of this report with her usual competence. The readability of the report benefited immensely from the exemplary editorial work of Andrea Posner.

Lastly, the chairman wishes to add that this report could not have been produced without the extraordinary efforts of Richard Rettig, who devoted more time, energy, and common sense to the effort than the committee and its chairman had any reason to expect or ask for. Neither could it have been produced without the active participation of committee members in the actual writing of the report—a practice that has characterized the Institute of Medicine from its beginnings—and in their willingness to resolve their differences in an amicable and reasonable fashion, making the task of the chairman that much less difficult.

> Adam Yarmolinsky, *Chairman*
> Committee on the Federal Regulation of
> Methadone Treatment

Contents

Federal Regulation of Methadone Treatment

Executive Summary

For nearly three decades, methadone hydrochloride (6-dimethylamino-4, 4-diphenyl-3-heptanone hydrochloride) has been the primary means of treating opiate addiction. Approved by the Food and Drug Administration (FDA) in 1947 for analgesic and antitussive uses, methadone was shown to be effective in treating opiate addiction in the mid-1960s and was approved by FDA for this use in late 1972. Pharmacologically, methadone is a weak-acting opiate agonist (that is, it imitates the action of an opiate, such as heroin) that does not generate the euphoria of an opiate but does reduce symptoms of opiate withdrawal. Today, an estimated 115,000 individuals receive methadone treatment for opiate addiction, and thousands more have benefited from it in the past.

The effectiveness of methadone treatment of opiate addicts has been established in many studies conducted over three decades. Methadone-maintained patients show improvement in a number of outcomes, after an adequate dose (usually 60–120 mg per day) is established. Consumption of all illicit drugs, especially heroin, declines. Crime is reduced, fewer individuals become HIV positive, and individual functioning is improved. These outcomes reflect the three objectives of methadone treatment: assisting the individual addict, enhancing public safety, and safeguarding public health. Outcomes serving these objectives are realized most often by the combined effects of the medication and the counseling provided by good treatment programs. The two factors limiting methadone's effectiveness are the multiple health and social problems of methadone maintenance patients, and the variability in quality of treatment programs.

HOW METHADONE IS REGULATED

Even though the effectiveness of methadone for treating opiate addiction has been well-established, its use has long been controversial, a fact reflected in its extensive regulation. First, the manufacturing, labeling, and dispensing of methadone are subject to the general requirements of the FDA for

1

establishing the safety, effectiveness, and consistent quality that are applied to virtually all prescription drugs under the Federal Food, Drug, and Cosmetic Act. Second, because methadone is a legal narcotic drug, its production, distribution, and dispensing are subject to the requirements applied to schedule II controlled substances by the Drug Enforcement Administration (DEA) to prevent diversion and illicit use.

In the case of methadone, a unique third tier of special standards has been established by the Department of Health and Human Services (HHS) prescribing how and under what circumstances methadone may be used to treat opiate addiction. These standards are implemented by FDA regulations, jointly with the National Institute on Drug Abuse (NIDA) since 1980 and, since 1993, with the Substance Abuse and Mental Health Services Administration (SAMHSA.) The FDA regulations issued in 1972 were designed to create a special "closed system" of distribution and use of methadone for opiate addiction treatment, restricted to hospital pharmacies and to physicians registered with both FDA and DEA who were authorized to dispense the medication in a treatment program only. This three-tiered system of federal regulation has continued for over 20 years and has recently been extended to a methadone analog, levo-alpha-acetyl-methadol (LAAM). The basic assumptions of this system have not been reviewed comprehensively during this period.

Methadone treatment of opiate addiction is often restricted still further by many state governments, a fourth level of regulation, a matter beyond the scope of this report. To complicate the picture even further, a fifth tier of regulatory authority over methadone treatment programs is sometimes found at the county and municipal level.

Two federal statutes require the Secretary of Health and Human Services to issue standards of treatment for narcotic addiction. Section IV of Title I of the Comprehensive Drug Abuse Prevention and Control Act of 1970 directs the Secretary to "determine the appropriate methods of professional practice in the medical treatment of the narcotic addiction of various classes of narcotic addicts." In addition, Section 3 of the Narcotic Addict Treatment Act (NATA) of 1974 required practitioners who dispensed methadone for maintenance or detoxification treatment to register each year with the Drug Enforcement Administration (DEA), which is instructed to register such applicants judged as qualified "under standards established by the Secretary" of Health and Human Services (originally Health, Education, and Welfare) to provide treatment services. Registrants are also required to comply with DEA's physical security and record-keeping requirements and with HHS's standards for "the quantities of narcotic drugs which may be provided for unsupervised use," namely, take-home medication.

SCOPE OF THE REPORT

The charge to the committee was to study current DHHS standards for narcotic addiction treatment and the regulation of methadone treatment programs pursuant to those standards. In this context, the committee sought to evaluate the effects of federal regulations on the provision of methadone treatment services and to explore options for modifying the regulations to encourage optimal clinical practice. It also considered the effects of the regulations on the development of new anti-narcotic medications, albeit briefly, as another IOM committee was convened to address this topic at length. Finally, it assessed the impact of the regulations relative to other factors affecting the provision of treatment services, and examined alternatives to the existing regulations.

In connection with the latter undertaking—examining alternatives to the existing regulations—a key point emerged concerning standards. Although the Secretary of HHS must set standards for narcotic addiction treatment, the sole means of doing so, historically, has been by federal regulations. But the implementation of standards *by regulations* is not required by law, and other options might be viable. In the course of developing this report, therefore, we examined alternative or complementary ways to implement standards, such as clinical practice guidelines and formal quality assurance systems (discussed on page 12 of this summary).

Although the study was limited to *federal* regulation of methadone, the report summarizes state rules in five jurisdictions—New York, California, Massachusetts, Illinois, and Florida. Unfortunately, a comprehensive description of the authorities and agencies of the states that govern opiate agonists used for treatment of opiate addiction does not exist. The limits of the charge and available data restricted the committee's evaluation of state regulation.

BALANCING THE BENEFITS AND RISKS OF METHADONE

Having completed its investigations, the committee urges reassessment of the appropriate balance between the risks of methadone and its benefits so that communities can attain the full potential benefit of this means of treating opiate addiction and its associated problems of crime, disease, and disorder, without increasing the risks of diversion and misuse. Current policy, in the committee's view, puts too much emphasis on protecting society *from* methadone, and not enough on protecting society from the epidemics of addiction, violence, and infectious diseases that methadone can help reduce.

Why, if methadone is effective, is it regulated so highly and so differently from other drugs? Three factors appear to have determined methadone's uniqueness as a regulated drug. First, methadone (and now LAAM), are the only opiates authorized for treating opiate-dependent persons. Thus, providing methadone to patients on a regular basis creates a potential for diversion and abuse. Second, the revision of regulations has been inhibited by inertia. Although the 1972 regulations were modified in 1980, 1989, and 1993, there does not appear to have been any major public effort to reexamine the underlying assumptions or long-term consequences of the regulations until this committee review was requested. Finally, neither public nor professional attitudes, nor those of the addict community, have supported methadone treatment strongly, and in the absence of this support the existence of federal regulations has provided local communities and society at large with assurance that their concerns about methadone were being addressed. In sum, the current regulations are predicated on a belief that the societal risks of methadone outweigh the societal benefits to such an extent that extraordinary controls are necessary above and beyond those applicable to any other therapeutic drug in the United States.

In the committee's view, this belief underlying the current regulations is not valid in today's environment and the regulations should be modified accordingly. The belief has its roots in the experience of the late 1960s and early 1970s, when knowledge of methadone was not extensive and the social risks associated with heroin use seemed largely confined to the addicts themselves. Today, however, we know much more about the risks and potential misuse of methadone. Although the drug can be abused, it is rarely a primary drug of abuse. Further, there is no apparent evidence of organized crime involvement in the street market for the drug.

At the same time, the committee finds that the current regulations produce unintended results: addicts who cannot obtain a treatment program tailored to their individual circumstances, physicians who are unable to exercise professional judgment in treating individual patients, programs that are isolated from mainstream medical care (thus depriving patients of important ancillary services), and significant economic costs in assuring compliance with regulatory requirements, costs that are shared by programs, insurers, patients, and taxpayers.

The committee has concluded that correcting these faults and, in general, raising the standard of treatment entails authorizing greater clinical discretion in medical treatment and reducing the scope of government regulation. There is no compelling *medical* reason, in the committee's view, for regulating methadone differently from all other medications approved by FDA, including schedule II controlled substances.

Nevertheless, the committee is not recommending abolition of the methadone regulations. Although, as stated above, there is no compelling *medical* reason for treating methadone differently, the committee recognizes that the regulations provide a number of positive benefits. The regulations address both a potential threat and a public fear of diversion. They help maintain community support for methadone treatment programs. They encourage comprehensive care and provide guidance to state authorities, hospitals, and medical practitioners. Although some believe that these latter goals can be accomplished by clinical practice guidelines alone, the committee believes that such guidelines, although necessary to guide practice, are not by themselves enough to assure that patients are cared for in a safe and thoughtful manner. Nor are they sufficiently developed at this time. **The committee concludes that a need exists to maintain certain enforceable requirements in order to prevent substandard or unethical practices that have socially undesirable consequences.**

In thus concluding that the regulations should be retained—but modified to give greater weight to clinical judgment, as determined by clinical practice guidelines—the committee considered one further aspect of the regulations. The regulations have been criticized as being "process-oriented"—imposing an undue administrative burden, infringing on clinical authority, and lacking any relationship to patient outcomes, program performance, and the quality of services provided. Although an "outcomes" approach might be useful, the committee believes that the current treatment system lacks the institutional infrastructure, including data systems, to support such a far-reaching step, a subject we return to below. Therefore, the committee recommendations to modify the regulations are ones that can be acted upon now, on the basis of existing empirical data. These recommendations include a number of changes in terminology, which emphasize that methadone and now LAAM involve the use of opiate agonist pharmacotherapy to treat opiate addiction, not the more pejorative and less descriptive "narcotic addiction," and that it is the addiction, not the addict, that is being treated. (All uses of narcotic in this summary and report refer to legal or official uses of the term, which is an unavoidable source of confusion.)

RECOMMENDATIONS TO MODIFY AND SUPPLEMENT THE REGULATIONS

The IOM committee developed the following general principles, according to which the regulations

- Should encourage that approved methadone programs make comprehensive care available to all opiate-addicted patients;
- Should emphasize the need for continuing clinical assessment of patients throughout treatment;

- Should provide clear instructions to programs regarding the procedures for the involuntary administrative withdrawal of medication, termination of treatment, or discharge of patients for whatever reason, and provide rights of due process to ensure safe and humane treatment;
- Should not arbitrarily restrict clinical practice;
- Should not promote withdrawal from methadone maintenance treatment without regard to the probability that the patient will return to opiate addiction;
- Should prohibit basing medication dose level on patient participation in or compliance with the treatment program.

In what follows, we describe some of the ways we applied these principles in recommending changes in the regulations (discussed in chapter 7).

Diagnosing Addiction and Determining Dose Levels

Regarding patient evaluation and admission criteria, the committee concluded that the assessment of opiate addiction **should be based on clinical diagnostic criteria and not set forth in regulations and that the diagnostic criteria for methadone pharmacotherapy should be set forth in clinical practice guidelines.**

With respect to dosing, which has long been controversial, current research findings and clinical experience can be summarized as follows: Patients vary in level of opiate tolerance and dependence, as well as in the absorption, metabolism, and elimination of methadone, and therefore it is necessary to determine each patient's dose individually. After initial dosing, the goal is to achieve full prevention of both signs and symptoms of withdrawal for 24 hours or longer, which requires that methadone "occupy" enough opioid receptors to prevent withdrawal; this may take a week or more and require further adjustments over time. The dose should both prevent withdrawal symptoms and reduce or eliminate drug hunger or craving. In some cases, assessing methadone blood levels may help to ensure adequate patient dosing in situations where patients have problems on doses that are usually in the therapeutic range. Pregnant patients are managed by the same general principles as maintenance pharmacotherapy, but with special considerations. **The committee recommends that the regulations retain the 30-mg limit on the initial dose to protect the safety of the newly admitted methadone patient, but that other dosing restrictions be removed from the regulations and made a matter of clinician judgment, augmented by clinical practice guidelines.**

Habilitative and Rehabilitative Services

The overriding goal of methadone maintenance treatment is to *habilitate* and *rehabilitate* patients with opiate problems to a basic level of social, work, and health capabilities and to help them become productive, independent members of society. Recent research about the rehabilitative goals of methadone maintenance treatment indicates, first, that opiate-dependent patients at the time of treatment admission typically display a wide range of serious medical, psychological, economic, and legal problems in addition to their opiate dependence. Second, these individuals show improvement in, if not elimination of, their opiate addiction with the provision of adequate doses of methadone. Third, improvements in the important social and self-support areas are at least partially related to the types and amounts of counseling and other social services provided during treatment.

The above research findings support the proposition that **the full potential of methadone maintenance as a significant public health service to society will be realized only if it is financially and professionally supported to the point at which it can offer necessary habilitative and rehabilitative services.**

Needed services include comprehensive evaluation of all patients admitted to methadone maintenance and medically supervised withdrawal; screening for AIDS, tuberculosis, hepatitis, and sexually transmitted diseases; on-site counseling by competent and appropriately supervised counselors; and professional medical, psychiatric, social work, and other mental health services. **The committee recommends that those services that are most clearly needed by admitted patients (e.g., medical, psychiatric, and social work) be provided on-site by competent, licensed, and appropriately supervised professionals wherever possible and, if necessary, by contractual referral arrangements.** The implementation of this recommendation requires that methadone maintenance treatment programs be restored to a level of funding and professionalism commensurate with the severity of the disorder(s) toward which they are directed. In the absence of such funding, however, a requirement to provide habilitative and rehabilitative services could very well impose an economic burden on many treatment programs that would force them to cease providing services at all.

Treating Pregnant Opiate Addicts

Although often complicated by confounding variables, research allows several favorable conclusions to be drawn regarding the usefulness of methadone pharmacotherapy in perinatal addiction, some of which follow:

Comprehensive methadone maintenance pharmacotherapy, when combined with appropriate prenatal care, can reduce the incidence of obstetrical and fetal complications, in utero growth retardation, and neonatal morbidity and mortality. There is no reported evidence of any toxic effects of methadone in the woman, fetus, or child. Withdrawal from methadone treatment is rarely appropriate during pregnancy, as relapse to illicit opiate use occurs in pregnant addicts in the same way as in nonpregnant or male addicts. Although neonatal withdrawal syndrome may occur in methadone-exposed neonates, treatment protocols are available to assist in appropriate patient management. On the basis of these and other conclusions drawn from research findings, **the committee recommends that regulations require that treatment programs establish rapid admission procedures to facilitate prompt treatment for pregnant opiate addicts; assure alternative ways to provide maintenance treatment for pregnant opiate addicts where treatment is not otherwise available; and allow providers to give maintenance pharmacotherapy for pregnant opiate addicts outside of a licensed narcotic treatment program, in settings such as a hospital, pharmacy, clinic, and individual practitioner's office. Special arrangements may be needed for patients in geographic areas where there are no licensed programs; dosage, treatment plan, and the acceptable time of treatment after conclusion of the pregnancy should be determined by consultation with addiction treatment experts, the treating physician, and the patient, in accordance with specific guidelines.**

Replacing "Detoxification" with "Medically Supervised Withdrawal"

Current regulations, based on the Narcotic Addict Treatment Act of 1974, specify arbitrarily defined treatment periods that bear no documented relationship to medical need or to clinical outcomes. Treatment based on these artificial time limits often results in the patient relapsing to illicit opiate use. Consequently, the committee is proposing that the regulations be changed to eliminate the term "detoxification treatment" and replace it with "medically supervised withdrawal," the principles of which are developed at length in chapter 7.

The outcome of medically supervised withdrawal is more likely to depend on personal motivation, patient resources, support systems (especially family), and appropriate comprehensive treatment than on the number of days in the withdrawal schedule. **Therefore, the committee recommends that the Narcotic Addict Treatment Act be amended, and the regulations changed, to eliminate the term "detoxification treatment" and replace it with "medically supervised withdrawal (MSW)"; that MSW be defined as the treatment of opiate dependence (using methadone or LAAM) that is** intended to achieve a zero dose over a treatment period that may range from a few days to perhaps six months, but that is not arbitrarily specified in the regulations; that regulations indicate clearly that MSW is not appropriate for all opiate addicts, but is an essential treatment that should be available to all who wish it or would benefit from it; and that clinical practice guidelines, based on the above general principles, be developed to assist clinicians in the clinical management of MSW patients, including the determination of appropriate dose schedules for individual patients.

Inpatient Hospital Admissions

Methadone patients admitted to hospitals as inpatients, whether for addiction-related reasons or for unrelated medical and surgical reasons, often are mistreated and mismanaged by hospital staff. This issue is appropriately addressed by guidelines for hospital staff, which should reflect the following general principles: on admission of a methadone maintenance patient as a hospital inpatient, hospital staff should notify the patient's treatment program and confirm the individual's enrollment, methadone dose, and time and date of last dose; during an inpatient stay, the hospital staff should ensure the continuity of methadone pharmacotherapy through its own pharmacy or by arrangement with the patient's treatment program; before discharge, hospital staff should notify the methadone treatment program of the time of discharge and the time and amount of last dose of methadone to ensure resumption of outpatient pharmacotherapy without interruption; if the patient is discharged to continuing care facilities, arrangements for continued provision of methadone should be part of the discharge plan.

In addition to the issue of how hospital staff care for methadone patients, there are problems of how the restrictions of the federal regulations affect the treatment of hospitalized opiate addicts in general. These restrictions may on occasion result in precipitous withdrawal of opiate-addicted patients. It may happen that admitted methadone patients do not receive methadone for opiate withdrawal relief because detoxification cannot be completed before discharge; or opiate-addicted inpatients may receive methadone treatment, but be precipitously withdrawn from methadone at discharge because transfer to an outpatient treatment program has not been made or existing programs have no capacity to accept them. The committee recommends that the regulations be changed to respond to the needs of hospitalized opiate-addicted patients so that patients who meet the criteria for opiate addiction during any inpatient hospital admission may be treated, as appropriate, with methadone to relieve opiate withdrawal; that they may then be discharged to methadone treatment programs for their continued treatment, or if no resources are available at discharge, or if a patient is ready for discharge before the withdrawal protocol can be completed, a hospital may complete the protocol on an outpatient basis; that a patient awaiting admission to a licensed narcotic treatment program may be maintained by the hospital on a maintenance dose of methadone until admitted by the program; that in all cases, methadone must be administered daily by hospital staff licensed to handle and administer narcotics; and that patients shall not be given prescriptions for methadone for these purposes.

Treating Opiate Addiction and Treating Pain

Methadone was approved by the FDA for the treatment of pain in 1947, but since the early 1970s it has been used primarily for the treatment of opiate addiction. There has been confusion about the two uses of methadone—treating opiate addiction and treating pain—that warrants clarification. Central to these issues is the need to distinguish the pain patient with no evidence of addiction from the opiate-addicted patient with chronic pain. The distinction to be made is that tolerance and physical dependence do not equal addiction. The patient with opiate addiction will seek drugs in the absence of any pain or withdrawal symptoms. The pain patient, on the other hand, will develop tolerance and physical dependence but will not exhibit the illicit or inappropriate drug-seeking behavior. The typical pain patient who experiences a cure or remission of pain does not experience the compulsion to resume or continue drugs.

The treatment of pain and the treatment of opiate addiction should be totally distinct. Although it may be appropriate occasionally to treat some pain patients in a methadone clinic, especially those that are an integral part of a hospital, it is not appropriate to treat a chronic pain patient *as an opiate addict* in a maintenance pharmacotherapy program. Similarly, persons suffering from opiate addiction are unlikely to receive appropriate treatment in pain clinics and, as a general rule, should not be treated for addiction in such clinics. Opiate addicts who also have chronic pain conditions may require coordinated treatment in both clinical settings, which sometimes may exist within in a single organization.

To address the problem of inappropriate referrals of pain patients—who may be opiate-dependent but not opiate-addicted—to methadone pharmacotherapy, **the IOM committee proposes that the regulations establish a clear distinction between opiate addiction and opiate dependence and that any guidelines developed for methadone treatment incorporate this distinction.** In addition, **the committee recommends that the regulations prohibit the** admission of a person being treated solely for chronic pain to an opiate addiction treatment program for treatment as an opiate addict. With respect to the problem of recovering opiate-addicted patients who experience acute pain and require opiate pain medication, on the one hand, such patients are often denied treatment for pain; on the other hand, these patients may in fact be at some risk for relapse to substance abuse or addiction, especially when the patient fails to inform the attending physician(s) of a history of alcohol or other drug use. Steering a course between these two dangers requires that medical staff serving opiate addiction treatment programs provide guidance to physicians, dentists, and other practitioners treating methadone-maintained patients for acute pain. In addition to emphasizing the need for honest communication between patient and physician, this guidance should provide for continued methadone pharmacotherapy without interruption; adequate doses of appropriate short-acting opiate agonist drugs for pain; and contraindications to giving antagonist and mixed agonist-antagonist opiate drugs that may produce a serious withdrawal reaction in opiate-tolerant individuals.

ENFORCEMENT OF THE REGULATIONS

The committee has drawn four conclusions about how the methadone regulations should be enforced (discussed in chapter 8):

First, the Drug Enforcement Administration should focus its attention on standards for the physical security and recordkeeping associated with the safe handling, storage, and dispensing of opiate medications (e.g., methadone and LAAM), as they do with other scheduled II drugs, but should have no role controlling or limiting medical practice.

Second, in response to the time-consuming, costly, and overlapping inspections of methadone treatment programs by federal, state, and, sometimes, county and municipal authorities, **the committee recommends that the FDA, with SAMHSA and NIDA, conduct an extensive review of the methadone enforcement policies, procedures, and practices of all health agencies of government—federal, state, and local—for the purpose of designing a single inspection format that would provide the basis for single, comprehensive inspections conducted by one agency that would serve all agencies and that would improve the efficiency of methadone service provision by reducing the number of inspections and consolidating their purposes.**

Third, to improve the competence of inspectors of methadone treatment programs, **the committee recommends that FDA, SAMHSA, and NIDA develop an annual training program for inspectors, whether from FDA,**

DEA, or state and local government agencies; that such a training program review all aspects of methadone treatment so that inspections are better focused and informed; and that this program be designed to support the consolidated review recommended above.

Finally, the committee believes that is necessary for an effective enforcement effort to close seriously deficient programs. The committee does not subscribe to the proposition that any program is better than none. An effective compliance program should close or bring into compliance substandard programs.

GUIDELINES AND QUALITY ASSURANCE

As stated above, the committee has concluded that the scope of federal regulation of methadone treatment should be reduced in favor of authorizing greater clinical discretion in determining appropriate medical treatment (see chapter 8). One means of assuring that clinical discretion is exercised in a sound manner is through clinical practice guidelines, defined by a 1990 IOM report (*Clinical Practice Guidelines*) as "systematically developed statements to assist practitioner and patient decisions about appropriate health care for specific clinical circumstances." Such guidelines are making their appearance in the substance abuse area, most notably in the Treatment Improvement Protocol (TIP) series of the Center for Substance Abuse Treatment (CSAT) of SAMHSA, and the committee considered them as a complete alternative to regulations. The committee concluded, however, that at this early stage of their development, guidelines are best employed as a complement, rather than a complete alternative, to existing regulations.

Formal quality assurance (QA) systems, either governmental or private, are another way to supplement reduced-scope regulations and shift responsibility for the provision of treatment services from regulators to clinicians. In the substance abuse area, formal QA systems are less well-developed than are practice guidelines. Designing a formal QA system involves selecting the outcome measures; devising instruments for measuring outcomes and for adjusting for severity of addiction and illness; and developing complex, valid data systems. The way substance abuse treatment is currently financed, no single revenue stream offers enough incentive to service providers to generate the requisite data. The Methadone Treatment Quality Assurance System, sponsored by NIDA, designed to assess the feasibility of a performance-based reporting and feedback system for methadone treatment programs, offers the prospect of laying the foundation for a formal QA system in the future.

PROCESS EVALUATION AND OUTCOME EVALUATION

Steps can be taken now, however, to set the stage for practice guidelines or QA systems (see chapter 8). In this connection, it needs to be pointed out that assessing quality requires process evaluation as well as outcome evaluation, and a way to relate the two. Process evaluation measures patient treatment procedures, which can be defined independently of the outcomes of care. For example, we suggest in the report that methadone maintenance patients be evaluated comprehensively for their medical, drug and alcohol, psychosocial, criminal, and employment problems; offered medical screening for AIDS, sexually transmitted diseases, tuberculosis, and hepatitis; given on-site counseling by well-trained and competently supervised professionals; and provided medical, mental health, and other social services, either on-site or by referral. These four processes could form the basis for QA process criteria standardized for clinical or administrative use by clinics or external evaluators.

While helping to assess whether therapeutic procedures are done "correctly" or not, however, process criteria do not indicate the effectiveness of the procedures. Effectiveness must be defined not only in relation to the individual well-being of the patient but also the public health and public safety objectives for methadone maintenance treatment, namely, the elimination of illicit opiate use and reduction of nonopiate illicit drug use; the general increase in positive social behaviors and employment; and the reduction of AIDS-transmission behaviors, crime, social violence, and the disproportionate use of medical and social services. We believe that the achievement of these objectives can and should be measured in any outcomes evaluation. Not every treatment program can by itself be expected to accomplish the full range of these objectives; achieving this goal will require integration and coordination with treatment services that may be provided by other agencies.

Outcomes can be objectively measured by medical and psychiatric examinations, evaluation of alcohol and drug use, verification of employment, and arrest records. Retention in treatment is a useful proxy measure of positive outcomes. The committee does not recommend that regulations be the vehicle for outcomes assessment; it urges instead that further steps toward instituting clinical practice guidelines and QA systems be taken.

FEDERAL GOVERNMENT LEADERSHIP

The need exists, in the judgment of the committee, for stronger federal government leadership in four areas: research, federal-state relations, the financing of substance abuse treatment, especially as it pertains to the use of methadone, and guidance on substance abuse treatment policy within the DHHS (see chapter 8).

There are two research issues on which the committee wishes to comment. First, it concurs in the conclusion of an IOM committee examining the NIDA Medications Development Program that the dual regulation by both FDA and DEA of clinical research in controlled substances is an unnecessary impediment to the conduct of such research (IOM, 1995). It endorses the recommendation of the other committee that "action be taken to remove the adverse effects of DEA requirements, under the Controlled Substances Act (CSA), on clinical research involving controlled substances, by holders of active FDA Investigational New Drugs (INDs), either by amending the CSA to exempt such IND investigations from applicable DEA regulations or by the alternative administrative and regulatory measures."

Second, the ADAMHA Reorganization Act of 1992 required that 15 percent of the research funds of the National Institute of Mental Health, the National Institute on Alcoholism and Alcohol Abuse, and the National Institute on Drug Abuse be spent in health services research. In the case of NIDA, compliance with this requirement will undoubtedly involve research on the delivery of substance abuse treatment services, some of which may involve methadone, LAAM, or other controlled substances. This research may involve such issues as treatment settings and take-home privileges.

Such health services research must be permitted to experiment with various institutional arrangements and not be subjected a priori to regulations that force it into a pattern prescribed by the methadone regulations. That is to say, if drug delivery in such research must comply with existing methadone regulations, we will never learn whether there are safer and more effective ways to treat addiction using alternative means of drug delivery, or whether these alternative means affect the potential for drug diversion and abuse. **The committee recommends that NIDA, in conjunction with SAMHSA, and FDA develop a general policy to guide health services research involving controlled substances such as methadone and LAAM, and negotiate a memorandum of understanding with the DEA to govern such research.**

With respect to federal-state relations, the committee notes that although federal regulations establish a common framework for methadone treatment services, there is great variation among the states regarding methadone treatment services. This variation stems from philosophical and financial factors that appear unrelated to the prevalence of opiate addiction and the characteristics of the treated patient population. (The report, in chapter 6, summarizes state rules in five states—New York, California, Massachusetts, Illinois, and Florida.)

In the course of examining the federal methadone regulations, the committee arrived at several general conclusions about the responsibilities of the federal government and the states.

First, a need exists to maintain a federal system of regulations that proscribe certain activities, such as using medication doses to reward or punish a patient's behavior, or failing to provide due process for involuntary administrative termination of treatment. In addition, clinical practice guidelines should be developed for methadone treatment, with state substance abuse authorities as a primary user.

Second, the federal government should actively attempt to minimize the administrative burden associated with both federal and state government regulation of methadone treatment. It should seek compatibility of federal and state regulations, and should adopt uniform procedures that allow inspections by one level of government to be satisfactory for other levels. It should, as appropriate, consider the delegation of the inspection and compliance function to the states on a contract basis.

Third, federal regulations should encourage states, through their licensing boards, to ensure that medical, psychiatric, nursing, psychology, social work, and pharmacy staff have adequate training to provide the appropriate care in methadone treatment programs.

Fourth, federal regulations should prohibit states that receive federal funding from developing regulations or contractual requirements that arbitrarily limit services and deny methadone pharmacotherapy to patients who require concurrent treatment for psychiatric illness and/or other addictions, or from arbitrarily limiting services even in the absence of such regulations or requirements. SAMHSA should be authorized and directed to tie compliance with this requirement to eligibility for block grant funding.

Finally, the extent of state regulation of substance abuse treatment revealed in the case of LAAM, approved by FDA in 1993 for treating narcotic addiction, but not yet approved by many states is so great that the committee recommends **that a comprehensive assessment of state substance abuse treatment regulations be undertaken, especially as they pertain to the treatment of opiate addiction, with an eye to developing a model state approach to the financing, treatment, and regulation of services.**

With respect to financing, the committee was not asked to examine this aspect of methadone treatment, and the descriptive data in chapter 6 do not permit any authoritative judgments to be made about the adequacy of financing. Recent evidence indicates, however, that there has been a marked decrease in the number and variety of services clients reported receiving. Although there are currently federal block grant monies to improve access to treatment, they do not appear to meet the current treatment demand. These and other financing limitations create serious barriers to treatment for many patients and limit the type and quantity of provided services.

The committee notes two developments pertaining to treatment financing. First, the fiscal year 1995 budget submission sent to Congress by President Clinton in early 1994 requested increased funding for drug treatment services relative to law enforcement activities. Second, the omnibus crime bill adopted by Congress in 1994 emphasizes prevention and treatment of substance abuse. It may be expected that increased federal funds will flow to substance abuse treatment services as a result of these actions. Therefore, the committee recommends **that DHHS conduct a review of its priorities in substance abuse treatment, including methadone treatment, in a way that integrates changes in regulations and the development of practice guidelines with decisions about treatment financing**.

With respect to drug abuse policy within the DHHS, current organization as revealed in the area of methadone, results in department policy emerging from the independent activities of the several pertinent Public Health Service agencies—SAMHSA, NIDA, and FDA—and from coordination between these agencies. The committee concludes that federal policy on methadone treatment, and in all likelihood broader areas of drug abuse treatment, would benefit from sustained *department-level policy oversight, informed by a clinical perspective*, on all issues related to regulations, practice guidelines, and treatment financing.

The committee does not believe that such a policy oversight role requires a major organizational change within DHHS, but that one official in the Office of the Assistant Secretary for Health should be designated to serve this function for the department. **The committee recommends that the Secretary of HHS direct the Assistant Secretary for Health to designate a senior official in the Office of the Assistant Secretary for Health to be responsible for policy oversight and guidance on methadone treatment and on related drug abuse prevention and treatment issues**.

REFERENCE

Institute of Medicine. 1995. Development of Medications for the Treatment of Opiate and Cocaine Addictions; Issues for the Government and Cocaine Addictions; Issues for the Government and Private Sector, CE Fulco, CT Liverman, and LE Earley, eds., National Academy Press, Washington, D.C.

1

Introduction

In the universe of addictions, opiate addiction, for which heroin is the primary drug of abuse, is and has been a major part of the general drug abuse problem. For nearly three decades, methadone has been the primary means of treating opiate addiction and its effectiveness for this purpose is well-established. Yet the use of methadone for the treatment of opiate addiction on a long-term (or maintenance) basis has been limited and controversial and remains so. This controversy is reflected in the fact that it has been regulated more extensively in this country than any other therapeutic drug.

Methadone, like all other prescription drugs, is regulated by the Food and Drug Administration (FDA) of the Department of Health and Human Services (HHS) under the Federal Food, Drug, and Cosmetic Act. Because it is classified as a narcotic drug[1] with some potential for abuse, methadone is also regulated like, other potent opiates, by the Drug Enforcement Administration (DEA) of the Department of Justice under the Controlled Substances Act. But

---

[1]"Narcotic" is defined by Stedman's *Medical Dictionary*, 25th edition, 1990, as "1. Any substance producing stupor associated with analgesia. 2. Specifically, a drug derived from opium or opium-like compounds, with potent analgesic effects associated with significant alteration of mood and behavior, and with the potential for dependence and tolerance following repeated administration. 3. Capable of inducing a state of stuporous analgesia." Legally, "narcotic drug" is defined by the Controlled Substances Act (21 USC 802 (17)) as "any of the following whether produced directly or indirectly by extraction from substances of vegetable origin, or independently by means of chemical synthesis, or by a combination of extraction and chemical synthesis: (A) Opium, opiates, derivatives of opium and opiates, including their isomers, esters, whenever the existence of such isomers, esters, ethers, and salts is possible within the specific chemical designation. Such term does not include the isoquinoline alkaloids of opium. (B) Poppy straw and concentrate of poppy straw. (C) Coca leaves, except coca leaves and extracts of coca leaves from which cocaine, ecgonine, and derivatives of ecgonine or their salts have been removed. (D) Cocaine, its salts, optical and geometric isomers, and salts of isomers. (E) Ecgonine, its derivatives, their salts, isomers, and salts of isomers. (F) Any compound, mixture, or preparation which contains any quantity of any of the substances referred to in subparagraphs (A) through (E).

unlike *any other* prescription drug and *any other* controlled substance, methadone—when used to treat opiate addiction—has *also* been subjected to a third layer of federal regulations. These regulations govern in great detail how physicians may—and may not—care for opiate-dependent patients and are enforced by federal agents.

The special methadone regulations flow from two statutory requirements that the Secretary of HHS (formerly the Secretary of Health, Education, and Welfare) issue standards of treatment for narcotic addiction. Section IV of Title I of the Comprehensive Drug Abuse Prevention and Control Act of 1970 (Public Law 91-513) charged the Secretary to "determine the appropriate methods of professional practice in the medical treatment of the narcotic addiction of various classes of narcotic addicts."

Section 3 of the Narcotic Addict Treatment Act of 1974 (Public Law 93-281) reiterated this authority and expanded the charge. It required practitioners who dispensed narcotic drugs to individuals for maintenance or detoxification treatment to obtain an annual registration from DEA. DEA was directed to register such applicants if, among other things, they were determined by the Secretary of HHS to be qualified "under standards established by the Secretary" to engage in the treatment activity.

Registration also required a determination by DEA that the applicant would comply with DEA's physical security and record keeping requirements and with HHS's standards, developed in consultation with DEA, regarding "the quantities of narcotic drugs which may be provided for unsupervised use by individuals in such treatment." "Unsupervised use" refers to take-home medication.

The focus of all these laws and regulations is a pharmaceutical agent. Methadone hydrochloride (6-dimethylamino-4, 4-diphenyl-3-heptanone hydrochloride) is a synthetic opiate developed in Germany during World War II as an alternative to morphine. It was approved by FDA in 1947 as a medication for analgesic and antitussive (relieving or preventing cough) uses.

In the mid-1960s, methadone was shown to be effective in the treatment of opiate addiction and thereafter became widely available for this use. Today, an estimated 115,000 individuals receive methadone treatment for opiate addiction, and many thousands more have received it over the past two decades.

There are two basic types of methadone treatment—detoxification therapy and maintenance therapy. *Detoxification therapy* involves the use of methadone to reduce the symptoms of acute abstinence (or withdrawal) following cessation of opiate use. *Methadone maintenance therapy* involves the use of methadone on a sustained basis to reduce or eliminate compulsive opiate use by substituting a drug that produces long-lasting activation of opioid receptors in the brain without causing uncontrolled craving effects or interfering with normal functioning in society. The term "methadone treatment" is used throughout this report to refer to the use of methadone (the drug) to treat opiate addiction, typically through a combination of dispensing medication *and* providing counseling and related health services.

THE CHARGE TO THE COMMITTEE

In 1992, the U.S. Public Health Service asked the Institute of Medicine (IOM) to evaluate the standards issued by the Secretary of HHS for narcotic addiction treatment pursuant to the 1970 and 1974 statutes and the regulation of methadone treatment programs pursuant to those standards. This is the report of the IOM committee convened to conduct that study.

The study was supported by the National Institute on Drug Abuse (NIDA) and the Center for Substance Abuse Treatment (CSAT) of the Substance Abuse and Mental Health Services Administration (SAMHSA). The FDA also participated in monitoring the study, and the Office of the Assistant Secretary of Health coordinated liaison between the project and these agencies.

The committee's view of the statement of work evolved over its first three meetings as it deliberated about the nature and purpose of the subject. Consequently, the committee revised its charge at its third meeting as follows:

> The committee will study the current Department of Health and Human Services standards for narcotic addiction treatment and the regulation of methadone treatment programs pursuant to those standards: (1) it will evaluate the effects of federal regulations on the provision of methadone treatment services and will explore options for modifying the regulations to encourage optimal clinical practice; (2) it will consider the effects of the regulations on the development of new antinarcotic medications; (3) it will assess the impact of the regulations relative to other factors affecting the provision of treatment services; and (4) it will examine alternatives to the existing regulations.

The above language then guided the committee through the duration of its study. It was subjected to a series of refinements of understanding as a result of the study process.

The principal departure of the revised charge from the initial work statement was to defer, without prejudice, the original suggestion for consideration of an "outcomes" approach to federal regulation. The methadone regulations have been criticized as being "process-oriented" and requiring compliance with administrative procedures that bear no relation to outcomes. Although an "outcomes" approach might be useful, the committee believes that the current treatment system lacks the institutional infrastructure, including data systems, to support such a far-reaching step. The committee's recommendations, therefore, are ones that can be acted upon now on the basis of existing empirical data; they are made in the interests of improving the current regulations. In addition, the committee has attempted to place the role of regulations and other instruments of public policy—clinical practice guidelines and formal quality assurance systems—in the context of more adequately fulfilling the responsibility of the Secretary for treatment "standards."

In approaching its charge, the committee limited the scope of the study to the special federal regulation of methadone, primarily to FDA regulations and to a lesser extent DEA regulations implemented under the authority of the Secretary of HHS to issue standards of treatment for narcotic addiction. Although the committee also examined how several state governments regulate methadone, it did not evaluate these regulations. Often state and local regulations impose significantly more severe constraints on the delivery of methadone treatment services than does the federal government.

OBJECTIVES OF OPIATE ADDICTION TREATMENT

The committee distinguished three objectives that guide the use of methadone in the treatment of opiate addiction. Although the relative importance of these objectives has shifted over time, the committee believes that all three should continue to inform policy.

The first objective of treatment is to reduce the severity of the addiction and the compulsive self-injection of heroin and thus allow the addict to establish or restore and maintain an acceptable level of medical and social functioning. Achieving this objective is complicated by the variability within the addict population with respect to simultaneous use of other addictive substances, other mental health problems, unattended medical problems (including HIV-related illnesses, sexually transmitted disease, multiple drug resistant tuberculosis, violence-related injuries, and malnutrition), low education, high unemployment, and weak family structure.

Heroin-addicted individuals are large consumers of costly emergency health care resources because they attend to their health needs on an episodic, crisis-oriented basis. Many are in poor health, and engage in high-risk behaviors that expose them to communicable diseases and violence. Moreover, they are often uninsured, and so do not attend to routine health problems. As a result, they often utilize hospital emergency services as their primary health care provider, which is costly and inefficient. When successfully treated with methadone, such individuals experience improved general health associated with a reduction in both drug use and high-risk behaviors. However, use of traditional medical resources remains difficult for these individuals, for these individuals, at least partly owing to real or perceived stigmatization of the addict and the methadone patient. On-site, or easily accessible and accepting, primary health care offers a solution to this problem.

If able to work, untreated heroin addicts are often so preoccupied with satisfying their addiction that they are unable to cope effectively with workplace responsibilities. By contrast, it is clear that many heroin-addicted individuals, when stabilized in methadone treatment programs, are able to obtain and maintain employment, develop access to health care resources and benefits, and care for themselves and their families.

The second objective of treatment is reducing crime and enhancing public safety. Treatment that removes individuals from consumption of illicit drugs also reduces criminal behavior motivated by the addict's need to support his or her drug purchases. Patients in methadone maintenance treatment programs have been shown to have markedly reduced criminal activity compared to their pretreatment behavior (Anglin and McGlothlin, 1985; Anglin and Powers, 1991; Anglin et al., 1989; Ball and Ross, 1991). Compared to drug-free treatment, methadone increases the likelihood of engaging and remaining in treatment, which is in turn correlated with the reduction of criminal activities.

The third objective of treatment is safeguarding public health, including the health of persons who do not abuse drugs, especially with regard to reducing the transmission of the HIV virus (which results in AIDS) and the transmission of other infectious diseases such as hepatitis and tuberculosis. This objective is served to the event that the at-risk addict population ceases or reduces intravenous injections of heroin, needle sharing, and sex-for-drugs transactions, and encounters physicians, nurses, counselors, and other public health workers who are able to treat a range of medical problems and reinforce healthy behaviors in an outpatient setting.

These three concerns—for individual functioning, public safety, and public health—provide the rationale for methadone treatment. They anchor the policy discussion in the recognition that multiple and competing objectives are being pursued. This recognition should help to achieve the appropriate trade-offs that lead to sound and effective public policy.

EFFECTIVENESS OF METHADONE MAINTENANCE TREATMENT

The effectiveness of methadone treatment of opiate addicts has been examined in many studies conducted over three decades. The early reports of Dole, Nyswander, Cushman, and others established the safety and pharmacological efficacy of methadone in the treatment of opiate dependence (Dole, Nyswander, 1968; Gearing, Schweitzer, 1974; Dole, Nyswander, et al., 1982). Since that time the clinical effectiveness of methadone maintenance has been evaluated in over 300 published reports (Hubbard, Marsden, et al., 1986; Sells, Demaree, et al., 1979). Even though there has been considerable variability in the methodology and results of these studies, the weight of evidence is that about 25–45 percent of opiate addicts who begin maintenance treatment continue successfully for a year or more (Hubbard, Marsden, et al., 1986; Sells, Demaree, et al., 1979).

Beneficial Outcomes

Once established on an adequate dose (usually 60–120 mg per day; see chapter 7 for discussion of dosing), methadone-maintained patients show improvement in a number of outcomes (Dole, Nyswander, 1968; Gearing, Schweitzer, 1974; Sells, Demaree, et al., 1979; Dole, Nyswander, et al., 1982; Hubbard, Marsden, et al., 1986). First, consumption of all illicit drugs declines. There are reductions in the frequency of heroin use to less than 40 percent on average of pretreatment levels during the first treatment year, as some addicts discontinue entirely, others reduce their use only slightly. Further reductions are achieved for patients who continue treatment for two or more years, eventually reaching 15 percent on average of pretreatment levels (Sells, Demaree, et al., 1979; Cummings, 1979; Newton, 1979; Rounsaville, Weissman, et al., 1982; Woody, Luborsky, et al., 1983; Khantzian, Treece, 1985; Wrangle, Corty, Ball, 1987; McNeil-Lehrer, 1988; Ball, Ross, 1993). In addition, crime is reduced, fewer become HIV positive, and individual functioning is improved.

Three studies discussed below illustrate these points, although several large-scale evaluations of methadone maintenance all show essentially the same results (Dole, Nyswander, 1968; Gearing, Schweitzer, 1974; Hubbard, Marsden, 1986; Sells, Demaree, et al., 1986; Ball, Ross, 1991). In the most detailed examination of methadone maintenance treatment programs to date, Ball and Ross (1991) showed that methadone maintenance was associated with significant reductions in illicit drug use and particularly crime. They evaluated twelve methadone maintenance programs in three northeastern cites, using two samples of newly admitted or stabilized patients, each sample obtained during 12 months over a five-year period.

Although there were differences in methadone treatment effectiveness as a function of the severity of the patient's condition, the number of services provided during treatment, and particularly the medication dose (larger doses producing better outcomes), the overall conclusion was that across all programs, methadone maintenance was associated with significant reductions in use of heroin and nonopiate drugs. There were also substantial reductions in crime from a rate of 237 crime days per year per 100 addicted persons during an average year of their addiction, to 69 crime days per year per 100 patients during the years of methadone maintenance—a reduction of over 70 percent from pretreatment levels. This is illustrated in Figure 1-1.

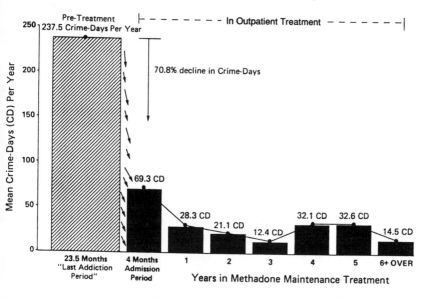

FIGURE 1-1 Reduction in crime by years in methadone maintenance treatment. SOURCE: Ball and Ross (1991), p. 205.

In a second study, Metzger et al. (1993) show the public health benefits of methadone treatment. They compared the rates of AIDS risk behaviors (particularly injecting drug use and needle sharing) between samples of opiate addicts in methadone maintenance treatment and those not in treatment. This study was interesting for two reasons. First, the two samples were recruited from the same neighborhoods and in fact the same groups social networks: patients in methadone maintenance were asked to refer friends and/or relatives who lived in the same communities and knew the same people, who had been using opiates at least three times per week, and who had been out of opiate treatment for at least the past year. Thus, the two samples were quite comparable with respect to histories of opiate use, demographic characteristics, and peer relationships.

In addition, this study followed both samples every six months for 36 months, achieving a 95 percent contact rate each time. Further, each follow-up evaluation included a blood test for HIV. Results were quite remarkable, as can be seen in Figure 1-2. At baseline, 13 percent of methadone-maintained opiate addicts were HIV positive, compared with 21 percent of the out-of-treatment opiate addicts. Over the following three years, an additional 5 percent of methadone-maintained opiate addicts became infected (interestingly, only those who dropped out of treatment). Among out-of-treatment opiate addicts, an additional 26 percent became infected over the same time period. These data do not prove that methadone was the causal agent generating the differences in infection rates, but they do suggest that participation in methadone treatment was at least one factor in the reduction of AIDS risk behaviors. This conclusion does not ignore the fact that self-selection by the treatment population may account for important differences.

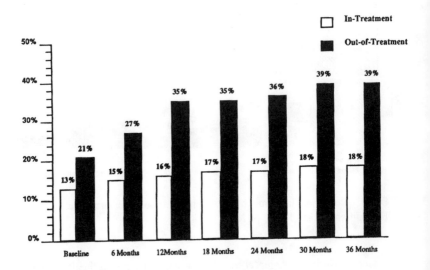

FIGURE 1-2 Three-year HIV infection rates by treatment status at time of enrollment. SOURCE: Metzger et al. (1993).

The third study evaluated the contribution of counseling and psychosocial services in methadone maintenance treatment, and shows the effect of these services on outcome. McLellan et al. (1993) randomly assigned newly admitted methadone maintenance patients, all of whom received basically the same methadone dose (the average dose was 65 mg/day and the range was 58–70 mg/day) to receive one of three levels of counseling and other services. (See also chapter 7.)

Level One patients received no other services except emergency counseling. Level Two patients received the same methadone dose plus standard contingency-based counseling.

In this group, patients' drug use was monitored by the counselor using weekly urine screenings. Patients who showed no drug use were not required to meet regularly while patients with positive urine screens were required to meet more frequently. No other services were provided. Level Three patients received the same counseling as the level Two patients but, in addition, had the availability of on-site medical care, family therapy, employment counseling, and psychiatric treatment.

Results of the six-month study indicated that level One patients did reduce their opiate use "as measured by urine screenings" but only by half as much as the other two groups. In fact, 69 percent of the level One group had eight consecutive positive urines. This was defined a priori as treatment failure and was used as a criterion for removing patients from the methadone-only condition and transferring them to standard treatment (i.e., methadone plus counseling). Only forty-one percent of level Two patients and 19 percent of level Three patients met this definition of treatment failure.

Figure 1-3 shows level One patients had the poorest outcomes in nearly all areas measured, especially in cocaine use, crime, and unemployment. Level Two patients showed significantly better outcomes than Level One patients in opiate and cocaine use and needle sharing. Level Three patients had significantly better outcomes than level Two patients relative to reduced cocaine use and needle sharing, and greater employment. These data indicate that although the dosage of methadone is extremely important and that adequate doses by themselves can produce significant reductions in pre-treatment levels of opiate use, greater reduction of heroin use was obtained through counseling and other services, and medication in conjunction with counseling and other psychosocial services produces much greater social rehabilitation.

These studies demonstrate the benefits of methadone maintenance. Still, two major factors limit its effectiveness. These are, first, the multiple health and social problems of methadone maintenance patients, and second, the variability in the quality of treatment program management and services.

Factors Limiting Effectiveness

Multiple Problems of Methadone Maintenance Patients

Although drug use (especially use IV drug) is the major focus of methadone treatment, it is only one of many complications seen in patients applying for methadone treatment. For example, studies by Rounsaville et al. (1982), Khantzian and Treece (1985), and Woody et al. (1983) have documented the high proportion of psychiatric diagnoses among methadone patients. Metzger and Platt (Ball, Ross, 1991; Metzger, Woody, et al., 1993) have shown the extreme frequency of unemployment and deficits in job-seeking skills among a large proportion of these individuals. Finally, studies by Stanton and his colleagues have documented the serious family and personal difficulties found in opiate-dependent patients being treated with methadone (McLellan, Arndt, et al., 1993).

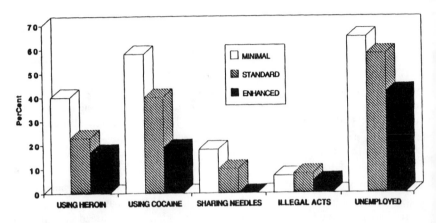

FIGURE 1-3 Methadone services: Target behaviors at six months by level of service. Minimal = methadone only, counseling in emergencies; standard = methadone plus standard counseling; and enhanced = standard plus psychosocial services. SOURCE: McLellan et al. (1993).

The multiple complexities of the methadone patient population significantly affect the course and overall results of treatment (Hubbard, Marsden, 1986; Sells, Demaree, et al., 1979; McLellan, Arndt, et al., 1993; Woody, McLellan, et al., 1987). For example, opiate addicts who have been stabilized by methadone maintenance but have experienced little improvement in their psychiatric, family, and employment situation will always remain in danger of relapse to injecting drug use. This of course has potentially large economic implications for any administrative decisions regarding the expansion of methadone treatment services. For example, a program of methadone maintenance alone, without counseling and other services, may be the least expensive way of effecting at least some improvement in drug use and AIDS-related behaviors. But, it is also possible that a more enhanced and expensive program, providing effective treatment for the medical, psychiatric, family, and employment difficulties of these patients, may be more cost-effective than the less expensive program in reducing AIDS related behaviors, encouraging rehabilitation, reducing crime, and controlling demands for welfare benefits and expensive medical services.

Variability among Methadone Maintenance Programs

The second factor limiting the effectiveness of methadone maintenance treatment is the variability among programs. Ball and Ross (1991) showed dramatic differences among methadone treatment programs in such fundamental outcome measures as proportion of opiate-positive urines and number of visits to the program. In general, the patients treated in these programs were quite similar in terms of their demographic characteristics and treatment problems at the time of admission to methadone maintenance across the different geographic sites surveyed. In contrast, the data gathered on the programs themselves revealed major differences in almost all areas of organization and service provision; and these program variables have been closely associated with patient outcome. For example, with respect to methadone dosage, one program had an average methadone dose of 20–25 mg while other programs averaged 55–60 mg per day. Moreover, the data show a clear inverse relationship between level of methadone dose and level of heroin consumption in the prior 30 days. Programs also differed sharply in the provision of access to medical care for their patients, use of ancillary psychotherapeutic medications (e.g., antidepressants and antipsychotics), uniformity of enforcement of rules, counselors' case loads, psychiatric input, quality of inservice training and physician facilities.

WHY METHADONE IS REGULATED DIFFERENTLY FROM OTHER DRUGS

If methadone is effective, why it is regulated so highly and so differently from other drugs? That question requires us to consider how it is actually regulated. First, the manufacturing, labeling, and dispensing of methadone are subject to FDA's general requirements for establishing the safety, effectiveness, and consistent quality of virtually all prescription pharmaceuticals. Second, because methadone is a narcotic, its production, distribution, and dispensing are also subject to the DEA requirements applied to schedule II controlled substances to prevent diversion and illicit use. These are the most rigorous requirements imposed on legitimate medicines that have a potential for abuse. Many useful and important therapeutic agents are subject to this dual system of control, including morphine, codeine, medicinal cocaine, amphetamines, and short-acting barbiturates.

In the case of methadone, however, a unique third tier of regulation is imposed: Special standards have been established prescribing how, and under what circumstances, methadone may be used to treat narcotic addiction (21 CFR 291.501 and 291.505). These standards are set and implemented by FDA, under authority vested in the Secretary of HHS. (Under a delegation of authority from the Secretary, FDA exercised its authorities in the issuance of regulations jointly with NIDA during the 1980s and, in 1993, with SAMHSA.) The regulations, issued by FDA in December 1972, were designed to create a special "closed system" of distribution and use of methadone, effectively restricting distribution to hospital pharmacies and to physicians registered with both FDA and DEA who could authorize dispensing of the medication in a treatment program only. This three-tiered system of federal regulation has continued for over 20 years and has recently been extended to a methadone analog, levo-alpha-acetyl-methadol (LAAM).

It is also essential to note that methadone treatment of opiate addiction is restricted still further by many state governments. Although a model uniform state statute for controlled substances abuse was promoted in the 1970s, individual states rejected or deviated from this model when enacting their own statutes in ways that permitted a fourth tier of regulation on use of methadone, often significantly more restrictive than federal regulation. The report summarizes state rules in five jurisdictions—New York, California, Massachusetts, Illinois, and Florida. Unfortunately, a comprehensive description of the authorities and agencies of the states that govern medications that may be used for treatment of opiate addiction does not exist. To complicate the picture even further, a fifth tier of regulatory authority over methadone treatment programs is sometimes found at the county and municipal level.

No other medication is so highly regulated. There are three basic reasons for this unique regulatory status. First, methadone (and, by extension, LAAM) is the only opiate authorized to be used to treat opiate addicts. Therefore, its intended use creates a potential for abuse different from that of other controlled substances insofar as providing methadone to patients on a regular basis creates special opportunities for diversion. The initial regulations were written in part, to respond to real abuses and to the perceived threat of diversion of methadone into illicit channels. For reasons spelled out below, the committee believes that the benefits both to the individual patient and to society at large from authorizing greater clinical discretion in methadone treatment far outweigh the risks from diversion, but we recognize the existence of both a real threat and considerable public fear of diversion.

Second, once regulations are adopted, bureaucratic inertia inhibits revision. Initially adopted in 1972, the regulations were modified in 1980, again in 1989, and changed twice in 1993. There does not appear, however, to have been any effort to reexamine the underlying assumptions or long-term consequences of the regulations, until this committee review was requested.

Third, there is the matter of attitudes. Neither public nor professional attitudes nor those of the addict community have provided strong support for methadone treatment. In this connection, the federal regulations have served function of providing local communities and society at large with some assurance that public and professional reservations about methadone were being addressed. In short, the regulations exist, in part, to garner support for methadone treatment.

The committee believes it is important to be realistic about the matter of attitudes if recommended policies are to be implemented effectively. We therefore expand somewhat on this point, as follows:

With respect to public opinion, a substantial segment of public opinion over the years has opposed the use of methadone for the treatment of opiate addiction, and another segment is ambivalent about its use. Public attitudes toward addiction of any type, but particularly heroin addiction, are overwhelmingly negative. The debate over the extent to which addiction is a disease or a moral failure remains unsettled in the public mind. The stereotypes of addicts are of individuals engaged in criminal activity, predatory toward others, and unable or unwilling to respect the norms of acceptable social behavior or participate in the work force. The public's fear of opiate addicts creates a reluctance to spend "treatment" dollars on them; it also creates sympathy for a criminal justice response.

Public attitudes have strongly affected the number and location of treatment clinics. The effort to open a methadone treatment clinic often arouses intense local opposition from the prospective neighbors, both poor and middle class. Instances abound of local community groups barring the opening of such clinics, and forcing clinics to close or move out of neighborhoods. In 1993, for example, a new methadone treatment program opened in New York was one of only three the state has opened in the last 20 years.

The attitudes of the public—and those of drug treatment professionals are also divided regarding the pharmacologic treatment of addiction on a maintenance basis. Negative attitudes towards maintenance pharmacotherapy are being tempered somewhat, the committee believes, by two factors. One is that few individuals in the general population have escaped some encounter with drug addiction, either in themselves or through a family member, friend, neighbor, or work-place associate. The other factor is that, over time, there has been a growing acceptance of the use of medications on a long-term basis for medical and psychological conditions as diverse as high blood pressure, chronic depression, or diabetes.

In general, members of the medical profession often share many of the negative attitudes of the general public. Many are either indifferent or hostile to its use for the treatment of heroin addiction. Ignorance about its effectiveness may stem from the fact that methadone maintenance historically has been poorly linked to the provision of primary and specialized medical care and to mental health services, both of which are often needed by patients.

To complicate matters still further, drug treatment providers themselves are often divided philosophically on the value of methadone maintenance. For example, an antagonistic relationship exists between methadone maintenance and those with a drug-free or substance-free philosophy. Indeed, the ranks of methadone treatment providers include those who support use of maintenance treatment and others who use methadone only for detoxification followed by drug-free therapies. These different approaches to treatment have not been reconciled, and are not easily addressed on strictly scientific grounds.

Finally, the addict population itself is ambivalent toward methadone treatment programs. Participation in methadone treatment involves a great loss of autonomy. The continued dependence on methadone makes the patient vulnerable to threats or actual withholding of the drug for valid or invalid reasons. Many addicts are unwilling to give up such autonomy until they reach a situation so desperate that they feel they have no choice. Others, especially those with jobs or other scheduled responsibilities, find it too burdensome to attend the clinic daily, as present regulations require.

THE COMMITTEE'S VIEW

The current regulations are designed to restrict distribution of methadone intended for therapeutic use, and to establish and enforce standards of medical care utilizing methadone, in order to prevent diversion of methadone into nonmedical channels and to exclude inappropriate persons from methadone treatment. In the committee's view, these regulations are predicated on a belief that the societal risks are so great, and the societal benefits so limited, that extraordinary controls are necessary above and beyond those applicable to any other therapeutic drug in the United States. This belief might have been valid and useful in the late 1960s and early 1970s, when experience with methadone was not extensive and the social risks associated with heroin use seemed largely confined to the addicts themselves.

Having studied the issues during a 18 month period (described below), the committee concludes that contemporary circumstances are dramatically different from those of 20 or more years ago. We know a lot more today about the risks and potential misuse of methadone. Although the drug can be abused, it is rarely a primary drug of abuse. Its therapeutic effectiveness has been clearly demonstrated, alone and in conjunction with other treatment activities. Untreated opiate addiction has been shown to be closely linked with other major public health and safety problems, including violent crime, AIDS, drug resistant tuberculosis, and hepatitis, disorders that can then jeopardize the health of those who have never used illicit drugs. Methadone treatment has been shown to reduce these health problems which are endemic in the addict community. Thus, methadone is no longer seen as a treatment designed to alleviate only the addict's problems, but also as a partial solution to a complex set of public health and safety issues.

In light of these considerations, the committee urges reassessment of the appropriate balance between the risks of methadone and its benefits. The current regulations foster situations where addicts cannot obtain a treatment program tailored to their individual circumstances, physicians are unable to exercise professional judgment in treating individual patients, programs are isolated from mainstream medical care (thus depriving patients of important ancillary services), and significant economic costs are incurred in assuring compliance with regulatory requirements—costs that are shared by programs, insurers, patients, and taxpayers.

We have concluded that there is no compelling medical reason for regulating methadone differently from all other medications approved by FDA, including schedule II controlled substances. Nevertheless the committee is not recommending abolition of the methadone regulations. The regulations serve important functions, not the least of which is to maintain community support for methadone treatment programs by assuring that the programs maintain standards and are subject to outside review.

What the committee does recommend is a careful readjustment of the regulatory controls so that communities can attain the full potential benefit of this effective means of treating opiate addiction and its associated problems of crime, disease, and disorder, without increasing the risks of diversion and misuse. In sum, current policy puts too much emphasis on protecting society from methadone, and not enough on protecting society from the epidemic of addiction, violence, and infections that methadone can help reduce.

REPORT ORGANIZATION

The report is organized around the questions that occupied the study committee. These questions pertain mainly to the use of methadone and, to some extent LAAM, for the treatment of opiate addiction. In addition, the use of methadone for analgesic purposes is discussed in Chapter 7 in the context of the unanticipated effects of the regulations on pain management. Chapter 2 begins by addressing the question "what is methadone?" describes the drug, the physiology of opiate addiction, and the pharmacology, safety, and rationale of the use of methadone in treating such addiction.

Chapter 3 presents an epidemiological perspective on the heroin addict population, the dominant group among opiate addicts, and deals with the characteristics of methadone maintained individuals, who are drawn from this larger pool. The chapter, in essence, asks, "Who are the direct beneficiaries of methadone maintenance treatment?" As indicated above, the committee believes that society—in terms of public safety and public health—benefits indirectly from the effectiveness of methadone in helping opiate addicts directly. The report sets forth the benefits of methadone treatment in this chapter and in chapter 2. Although chapter 3 presents extensive data on New York and California, the scope of the research informing the study and the committee members' own knowledge and experience was far broader.

In chapter 4, the risks of diversion of methadone are discussed. The attention devoted to this subject derives from the fact that concern for diversion has loomed large historically and continues to play an important part in policy discussions about the use of methadone for opiate addiction treatment.

The manner in which methadone is regulated, that is, the way in which the balance has been struck between the benefits and risks of methadone treatment, is addressed in chapter 5. Historically, treatment standards have been implemented by exclusive reliance on regulations; the chapter describes the evolution of the current regulations.

Chapter 6 examines how methadone treatment is being delivered today. Attention is given to the providers of treatment, to treatment financing, and to the activities of five state substance abuse agencies.

Chapter 7 presents the changes the committee believes should be made in existing regulation to improve treatment. To describe the characteristics of good treatment, the chapter focuses on clinical concerns such as access to treatment, comprehensive services, adequate dosing, integration with primary care and other social services, flexibility to respond to changes in drug use within the patient population and to changing requirements for service intensity of individual patients, and respect for patient rights.

Chapter 8 examines alternative ways that standards might be implemented. These ways include regulations and the associated issues of enforcement, clinical practice guidelines and formal quality assurance systems. The chapter also considers federal leadership in research, federal-state relations, financing, and policy guidance. The committee emphasizes that it is not enough simply to recommend changes in the regulations without also addressing these interrelated issues of funding, access, quality assurance, mainstreaming of care, and greater acceptance of methadone maintenance treatment by insurers, the medical community, politicians, and the public. Regulations are not sufficient to ensure good service delivery or good medical care for patients; other commitments are necessary.

STUDY METHODS

The committee used a number of approaches to inform itself about the issues in this study. It met five times over a eighteen-month period to hear presentations by government officials, to give its members an opportunity to report on their own experiences, and to discuss the issues raised in this volume. All meetings, save the last, were two days in length. Project staff and a number of committee members attended the National Methadone Conference of November 1992 in Orlando, Florida, and the National Methadone Conference of April 1994 in Washington, D.C. The latter afforded an opportunity for approximately half of the committee to hold a brief evening meeting—the "sixth," strictly speaking. Except for this last occasion and the fifth meeting, all meetings, were open and were attended by representatives of the government agencies involved and other interested parties.

The committee chairman and several members attended and participated in the June 1993 meeting of the College on Problems of Drug Dependence, in Toronto. Site visits involving committee members and project staff were made to methadone clinics in Washington, D.C., Baltimore, New York, Boston, and Cambridge, Massachusetts.

In addition, half-day meetings were held between a small group of IOM committee members and IOM staff and representatives of various government agencies. One such meeting was with the staff of the FDA's inspection, compliance, and enforcement effort to familiarize the committee with these aspect of the regulations. Another such meeting was held with representatives of the DEA. This meeting, in turn, resulted in a subsequent visit to DEA offices by the IOM study director for follow-up information. A third meeting was held with the officials of the NIDA Medications Development Division. Project staff also had regular interaction with officials of NIDA, SAMHSA/CSAT, FDA, and DEA. The committee chairman and the study director met once with Mr. Peter Edelman, Counsel to the Secretary of HHS responsible for substance abuse policy, and once with Dr. Lee Brown, Director of the Office of National Drug Control Policy.

One paper was commissioned, which became the basis for chapter 6. Computer runs of data used in chapters 3, 4, and 6 were provided to the committee by the Drug Use Forecasting group of the National Institute of Justice, of the Department of Justice, by the Community Epidemiology Branch of NIDA, by the Office of Applied Studies of SAMHSA, and by the New York Office of Alcoholism and Substance Abuse Services. A series of special computer runs dealing with heroin addiction were performed using the data of the Epidemiological Catchment Area study, arranged by Dr. Lee Robins, a committee member.

Visits by the study director, accompanied by one or several committee members, to New York and Boston resulted in meetings with methadone program administrators in these states. The IOM requested that the New York Committee of Methadone Program Administrators (COMPA) provide it with a commentary on the regulations, which COMPA did to the committee's great benefit. Similarly, through Commissioner Marguerite Saunders, of the New York Office of Alcoholism and Substance Abuse Services, and a committee member, the state methadone authorities were asked for comment and complied in about half the cases.

A NOTE ON TERMINOLOGY

As chapter 3 in this report points out, there is no official psychiatric diagnosis termed "opiate addiction," and instead Diagnostic and Statistical Manual of Mental Disorders, Fourth Edition (DSM-IV), offers four related diagnoses: opiate dependence, opiate abuse, opiate intoxication, and opiate withdrawal; several symptoms whose presence may warrant a diagnosis of dependence, according to DSM-IV, are described. A detailed definition of addiction may be found, however, in Dorland's *Medical Dictionary*, as chapter 3 also points out; this definition specifies four symptoms that are characteristic of addiction.

Notwithstanding these and other variations to be found among contemporary authoritative sources, this committee employs the concept of addiction and related concepts, as follows:

Addiction is a condition distinguished by a lack of control and compulsion that leads to illicit or inappropriate drug-seeking behavior. It can occur with or without physical dependence. Opiate addiction has been operationally defined as at least one year of daily repeated opiate self-administration, with development of tolerance, physical dependence, and drug-seeking behavior (see chapter 2). Chapter 3, whose purpose is to describe the recipients of methadone treatment, lays stress on that aspect of addiction whereby the addict finds it impossible to stop using opiates without help.

Tolerance is the condition that results from continued use of an opiate drug (or of any substance) and that makes it necessary to use increasing amounts of the drug to produce the desired physiological and psychological effect.

Physical dependence results from repeated use of a drug, such as an opiate; the physiological systems adapt to such use to the point that they actually require the drug just to maintain physiological equilibrium. Although physical dependence is associated with tolerance, the latter can occur without causing physical dependence. The withdrawal symptoms associated with dependence are described in chapter 2.

An important distinction made in this report is that tolerance and physical dependence do not equal addiction. Chapter 7 discusses this distinction and the related definitions, and in addiction defines several other terms that belong to the lexicon of methadone treatment.

Finally, another distinction made in this report is between the terms "narcotic" and "opiate." Because "narcotic" refers to a stupor-inducing drug and is a legal term that includes cocaine (see detailed footnote earlier in this chapter), the committee reserves its use for discussion having a legal or statutory context. In all other discussion we use the term "opiate." The committee finds the distinction an important one and incorporates it into its recommendations.

REFERENCES

Anglin, MD, and McGlothin, WH. 1985. Methadone maintenance in California: A decade's experience. In L. Brill and C. Winick (eds.), *The Yearbook of Substance Use and Abuse* 3:219–280.

Anglin, MD, and Powers, KI. 1991. Methadone treatment and legal supervision: individual and joint effects on the behavior of narcotics addicts. *Journal of Applied Behavioral Science* 27(4):515–531.

Anglin, MD, Speckart, GR, Booth, MW and Ryan, TM. 1989. Consequences and costs of shutting off methadone. *Addictive Behaviors*, 14:307–326.

Ball, JC, and Ross, A. 1991. *The Effectiveness of Methadone Maintenance Treatment: Patients, Programs, Services, and Outcomes.* New York: Springer-Verlag.

Comments of Representative Rangle C (D-NY). 1988. McNeil-Lehrer Report, Public Broadcasting System (February 9).

Corty, E and Ball, JC. 1987. Admissions to methadone maintenance: Comparison between programs and implications for treatment. *Journal of Substance Abuse Treatment* 4(3):181–187.

Cummings, N. 1979. Turning bread into stones: Our modern anti-miracle. *American Psychologist* 34:276–239.

Dole, VP, Nyswander, M. 1968. Successful treatment of 750 criminal addicts. *Journal of the American Medical Association* 206:2708–2710.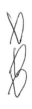

Dole, VP, Nyswander, M, and DesJarlais D. 1982. Performance-based rating of methadone maintenance programs. *New England Journal of Medicine* 306:169–172.

Gearing, FR and Schweitzer, MD. 1974. An epidemiological evaluation of long-term methadone maintenance. *American Journal of Epidemiology* 100:101–105.

Hubbard, RL and Marsden, ME. 1986. Relapse to use of heroin, cocaine and other drugs in the first year after treatment. In *Relapse and Recovery in Drug Abuse.* NIDA Research Monograph 72, USGPO, Rockville, Md.

Khantzian, EJ and Treece, K 1985. DSM-III psychiatric diagnosis of narcotic addicts. *Archive of General Psychiatry* 42:1067–1071.

McLellan AT, Arndt LO, Woody GE, Metzger D. 1993. Psychosocial Services in Substance Abuse Treatment? A dose-ranging study of psychosocial services. *The Journal of the American Medical Association* 269(15):1953–1959.

Metzger DS, Woody GE, McLellan AT, Druley P, DePhillips D, O'Brien C, Stolley P and Abrutyn E. 1993. HIV seroconversion among in and out of treatment intravenous drug users: An 18-month Prospective Follow-up. *AIDS* 6(9):1049–1056.

Newton, J. 1979. Methadone promise is unfulfilled. *Journal of Drug/Alcohol Abuse* (December 1):1–2.

Rounsaville, BJ, Weissman, MM, Wilber, CH. 1982. The heterogeneity of psychiatric diagnosis in treated opiate addicts. *Archive of General Psychiatry* 39:161–166.

Sells, SB, Demaree, RG and Hornick, CW. 1979. Comparative Effectiveness of Drug Abuse Treatment Modalities, NIDA Services Research Administrative Report, Washington, D.C.

Woody GE, Luborsky L, and McLellan AT, et al. 1983. Psychotherapy for opiate addicts: Does it help? *Archive of General Psychiatry* 40:639–645.

Woody, GE, McLellan, AT, Luborsky, L, et al. 1987. Psychotherapy for opiate dependence: A 12 month follow-up. *American Journal of Psychiatry* 145:109–114.

Woody, GE, McLellan, AT, Luborsky, L, et al. 1984. Severity of psychiatric symptoms as a predicator of benefits from psychotherapy: The Veterans Administration-Penn Study. American Journal of Psychiatry 141:(10)1172–1177.

2

Pharmacology and Medical Aspects of Methadone Treatment

Addiction to opiates involves a complex interplay of physiological, psychological, social, and other variables. The primary purpose of methadone treatment is to intervene directly in the physiological processes that underlie addiction. Ideally, such treatment is supported by additional psychological and behavioral therapies. To understand why methadone treatment works, it is important to understand the physiological basis of heroin addiction.

This chapter provides an overview of the development of pharmacotherapeutic approaches to the treatment of opiate addiction and summarizes the key basic scientific investigations of the physiological underpinnings of opiate effects, including the discovery of the endogenous opioid system. In addition, the chapter describes the pharmacological and medical characteristics of methadone as a medication for the treatment of opiate addiction.

THE RATIONALE FOR PHARMACOTHERAPY

History and Practice

Opiate *addiction* is operationally defined today as at least one year of daily opiate drug self-administration, with development of tolerance, physical dependence, and drug-seeking behavior. The concepts of *tolerance* and *dependence* are thus fundamental to understanding the physiological aspects of opiate addiction. When a person repeatedly uses an opiate drug like heroin, over time, that person becomes tolerant to heroin; that is, he or she requires greater and greater doses of heroin to achieve the same physiological and psychological effects. The same is true for the opiate drug morphine. Tolerance can be thought of as an adaptation of the functional (physiological) systems of the body to opiates. During chronic use of an opiate, physical dependence also develops when the physiological systems have adapted to the point that they actually require the opiate just to maintain physiological equilibrium.

Virtually all physiological systems are affected in opiate addiction. A reproducible syndrome occurs when an opiate addict goes through withdrawal. This syndrome includes yawning, lacrimation, piloerection, perspiration, mydriasis, tremor, gooseflesh, restlessness, myalgia, anorexia, nausea, vomiting, abdominal cramps, diarrhea, fever, hyperpnea, and hypertension. When prolonged, the syndrome includes weight loss and, even after acute withdrawal, symptoms subside, persistent symptoms such as sleep disturbances, irritability, restlessness, and poor concentration which can be present for months or years. Both acute and chronic tolerance are physiological phenomena subserved by the central nervous system. However, both acute and chronic tolerance may also be influenced by environmental variables, such as setting, conditioning, and learning.

The pharmacological approach to long-term treatment of heroin addiction, first undertaken in early 1964, was rooted in what was then a hypothesis that opiate addiction is a metabolic disease, caused by either intrinsic or drug-induced alterations in physiology. The original researchers in the field, Drs. Vincent Dole, the late Marie Nyswander and Mary Jeanne Kreek, hypothesized that in some or most cases of heroin addiction the addicted individuals had a intrinsic metabolic disorder, possibly with an underlying genetic predisposition, which expressed itself clinically after initial exposure to specific types of drugs or other chemical agents of abuse; and that in other cases, individuals who developed addiction were experiencing drug-induced metabolic disruptions in otherwise normal physiology. They speculated that in the latter cases, heroin-induced changes in specific neurobiological systems persist over long periods and possibly become permanent.

The researchers observed that gradual removal of physical dependence upon morphine or heroin (detoxification) followed solely by psychiatric or other behavioral treatment frequently failed to help addicts sustain abstinence. Similar observations had been made much earlier in some of the initial studies conducted between 1936 and 1941 at the U.S. Public Health Service (USPHS) Hospital in Lexington, Kentucky, which showed that less than ten percent of "hard-core" addicts were able to stay free from opiates after discharge from long stays in drug-free treatment programs that only offered counseling and psychiatric care.

Thus, Dole, Nyswander, and Kreek sought an optimal pharmacological agent that could supplant or complement psychological and behavioral treatment approaches. Their first study in 1964 was to repeat earlier studies that attempted unsuccessfully to use short-acting opiates, such as heroin and morphine, in a controlled fashion, in the management of opiate dependence. Morphine was again shown to be an unsuitable pharmacotherapeutic agent for several reasons: short duration of action, requiring four to six administrations per day; necessity for parenteral administration, because of lack of substantial bioavailability after oral administration; and the rapid development of increasing tolerance. Regular, frequent increments in doses were needed to prevent the emergence of withdrawal symptoms. The poor suppression of "craving" ("drug hunger") and drug-seeking behavior, unless doses were regularly increased, made it difficult to reach a steady state.

In view of the anticipated limitations of morphine as a maintenance agent, a search was made for a medication that would block withdrawal symptoms of heroin addicts and that would be orally effective, long-acting, nonsedating, and devoid of adverse side effects. Methadone, a synthetic opiate compound originally synthesized in Germany for use as an analgesic in World War II, was selected for study in 1964. Methadone had been introduced between 1958 and 1962 at the USPHS hospital in Lexington, at the Bellevue Medical Center in New York City, and at a limited number of other sites for "detoxification" treatment of heroin addiction. In the early detoxification programs it was given in three or four small daily doses, usually 5 to 10 mg each, because the prolonged duration of action was not yet appreciated and no analytical techniques existed for objective measurements of pharmacokinetics. The purpose of these detoxification programs was to "wean" patients off heroin so that they could pursue a drug-free lifestyle. However, these efforts largely failed. Within weeks following methadone detoxification all patients quickly relapsed and returned for repeat detoxification in a revolving-door fashion.

Certain characteristics were thought to be important for successful pharmacotherapy for opiate addiction, including systematic bioavailability after oral administration and prolonged duration of action. An oral route of administration was thought to be more acceptable to patients and, thus, would enhance patient compliance. Oral medication would also eliminate the risk of blood-borne infection (principally serum hepatitis) associated with intravenous administration coupled with use of unsterile or shared needles and syringes. Lastly, oral administration would disrupt the symbolic linkage to an illicit lifestyle and, practically, diminish the behavior of congregating to share needles and other drug paraphernalia.

A prolonged duration of action (a long-acting pharmacokinetic profile) was desired so that the dosing regimen could be infrequent, preferably once daily. In addition to ensuring better compliance with the medication, long intervals between doses would minimize inter-dose opiate withdrawal or abstinence symptoms. It was hypothesized that such a long-acting pharmacokinetic profile would also permit normalization of specific physiological functions disrupted by chronic use of short-acting opiates such as heroin. It was further hypothesized, and later proven, that long-acting agents would be effective at a stable dose for a much longer period of time owing to slower development and sustained level of tolerance. In fact, subsequent studies have shown that once the daily dose of methadone has been stabilized, tolerance does not develop to the essential effects of methadone (prevention of opiate abstinence symptoms and prevention of drug hunger or craving) as used in maintenance treatment. Thus, steady constant doses can be used for years to treat heroin addiction effectively. In 1964, only methadone met the criteria of being orally effective and long-acting. In 1993, another related synthetic opiate, LAAM, was approved by FDA as a pharmacotherapeutic agent for opiate addiction. LAAM has an even slower onset of action than methadone and more prolonged duration of action.[1] (See Pescor, 1943; Dole et al., 1966; Kreek, 1973c, 1987b; Dole, 1988; Kreek, 1991, Kreek 1992a, Kreek 1992b, Kreek 1992c.)

Basic Science

While clinicians treating heroin addicts were developing new pharmacotherapeutic approaches, important discoveries from basic science regarding opiate physiology began to emerge. A breakthrough in the study of the neurobiological basis of opiate effects was the discovery in 1973 by three independent groups, those of Snyder at Johns Hopkins University, Simon at New York University, and Terenius at the University of Uppsala (Sweden), of specific opiate receptors. These studies revolutionized the field of neuropharmacology and neurochemistry and were based, in part, on the earlier work of Dole and Goldstein. Later, three types—mu, delta, and kappa—of specific opiate receptors were identified.

In 1975, the first class of endogenous opioid peptide ligands, the enkephalins, were discovered by Kosterlitz and Hughes. Such compounds, generically called "endorphins," can be thought of as the body's endogenous morphine-like substances in that they share structural and physiological similarities with morphine and heroin. Soon thereafter, attention focused on three separate classes of endogenous opioid ligands that bind to the specific opioid receptors. In animals, many of the well-known opiate effects have been reproduced by administering large amounts of these endogenous opioids.

---

[1] This pharmacologic effect depends primarily on the metabolism of the parent LAAM compound to two active metabolites, noracetylmethadol and dinoracetyl-methadol. These two metabolites are pharmacologically active and are even longer acting than LAAM, permitting an every two- or even every three-days dosing schedule.

Tolerance develops to some of these natural opioid peptide effects. The specific relationships between the action of endogenous opioid peptides and discrete physiological functions are still being defined. Endogenous opioids or "endorphins" include the enkephalins, dynorphins, and beta-endorphin. The three opioid peptide genes have been cloned, and each encodes a single large peptide, which is then processed to yield all of the opioid peptides within a class: proenkephalin, prodynorphin, and proopiomelanocortin, the latter of which contains both beta-endorphin and other important nonopioid peptide hormones including adrenocorticotropin hormone (ACTH). As mentioned above, there are at least three types of specific opiate receptors, mu, delta, and kappa, each of which may have several subtypes. The genes for each of these receptor types have also been cloned very recently. Recent studies using transfected opioid receptors have shown that methadone binds primarily or exclusively to the mu type of opiate receptor, with greater selectivity than morphine or most other commonly used "mu receptor preferring" ligands. Currently, studies are in progress to localize and characterize gene expression of the endogenous opioid system peptide and receptor genes, to assess the effects of drugs of abuse and treatment agents on gene expression, and to understand the complex molecular biological interactions of this system.

Both basic and clinical studies have focused on the possible role of the endogenous opioid system in the biological basis of addiction. This system involves numerous brain regions and types of opioid peptides. Although the complex interactions of this system within the brain are not fully understood, data suggest that cycles of heroin addiction severely disrupt this system and that chronic, steady-state methadone maintenance attenuates this disruption. A "metabolic disease" concept has been suggested, in addition, which holds that some individuals may be predisposed to heroin addiction because variations in their genes result in abnormal levels of endogenous opioid peptides, levels that can be "corrected" by taking heroin (Goldstein, 1994). The effect of heroin addiction on the genetic regulation of the endogenous opioid system is currently an active area of research that is beginning to reveal intriguing clues about the biological underpinnings of addiction.

Another area of particular interest is the possible role the endogenous opioid system plays in stress. It has been hypothesized that an atypical responsivity to stress, including the common stresses in our daily environment, may contribute to the acquisition of drug-seeking behavior, and both laboratory and basic clinical research studies have been conducted to define the stress responsive axis in humans with addictive diseases and in animal models. One of the most important modulators of stress responsivity is the hormones of the hypothalamic-pituitary-adrenal axis. It is known that a peptide hormone released from the hypothalamus, corticotropin releasing factor (CRF), drives the anterior pituitary in humans to release peptides from one important gene product, proopiomelanocortin (POMC), which yields both the long known peptide hormone ACTH and as one of the endorphins, beta-endorphin. ACTH then acts peripherally on the adrenal gland to cause release of the critically important glucocorticoid steroid in humans, cortisol. In addition to many peripheral actions, cortisol acts in a negative feedback control manner to control both CRF release from the hypothalamus and the release of POMC peptides, ACTH, and beta-endorphin, from the anterior pituitary in humans. Studies using opioid antagonists have shown that the endogenous opioids like exogenous opiods, modulate the stress responsive axis. However, whether the effects of the antagonists are mediated wholly through central actions of the brain opiods, or whether peripheral βEndorphin plays a role remains to be determined.

(See Dole, 1970; Ingoglia and Dole, 1970; Goldstein et al., 1971; Kreek, 1973a, Kreek, 1973c; Pert and Snyder, 1973; Simon et al., 1973; Terenius, 1973; Hughes et al., 1975; Kreek, 1978b; Kreek and Hartmen, 1982; Kreek, Schaefer, et al., 1983; Kreek, Wardlaw, et al., 1983; Kreek, Raghunath, et al., 1984; Kreek, Schneider, et al., 1984; Kreek, 1987a; Branch et al., 1992; Evans et al., 1992; Hurd et al., 1992; Kiefer et al., 1992; Kreek, 1992c; Chen et al., 1993a, 1993b; McGinty et al., 1993; Spangler et al., 1993a, 1993b, 1994; Wang et al., 1993; Yasuda et al., 1993; Unterwald et al., 1993; Kreek, Simon, et al., 1994; Spangler et al., (in press.)

PHARMACOKINETICS OF METHADONE

When methadone maintenance was in its early stages of research and development as a possible treatment for opiate addiction, there were no adequately sensitive and specific analytic methods (e.g., gas-liquid chromatography, mass spectrometry, high-performance liquid chromatography or radioimmunoassay techniques) with which to assess the pharmacokinetics of methadone (or any other opiate such as morphine and heroin); that is, the time course of distribution, metabolism, and clearance in the body. Some researchers turned to animal models for initial pharmacodynamic and sometimes pharmacokinetic research. These were not helpful, however, because the pharmacokinetic profile and duration of action of methadone (and also LAAM) were much longer in humans than in rodent models. Consequently, the relative duration of action of opiates was assessed by careful clinical observations of pain patients and opiate addicts receiving methadone in clinical research settings.

Both morphine-induced analgesia in pain patients and euphoria in opiate addicts have a rapid onset and decline; within 4–6 hours, another dose is required. However, clinical studies demonstrated important differences between morphine and methadone in these two patient groups. Although in early studies methadone seemed to provide full analgesia for only 4–6 hours in pain patients, similar to morphine, when repeated doses of methadone were given over 24 hours, opiate-like side effects were observed. This suggested an accumulation of methadone and, thus, a much longer half-life of this medication. When methadone was given to heroin addicts, it seemed to prevent signs and symptoms of withdrawal for 24 hours. During oral administration of methadone to opiate addicts on doses selected to be less than those to which tolerance had been developed, the "high" or euphoria, and all other perceived opiate effects, are minimal or even absent.

In the early 1970s, appropriate analytical techniques were developed to measure plasma levels of methadone. These techniques substantiated the early clinical observations and showed that there was a gradual onset of action of orally administered methadone and that low peaks of methadone were reached. Peak plasma levels were usually less than twice the trough levels, and relatively steady-state sustained plasma levels of methadone were maintained during the remainder of the 24-hour dosing interval. The mechanisms that maintain the steady-state plasma levels were shown to include binding of methadone in body tissues (primarily the liver), with subsequent release into the circulation, and extensive plasma protein binding, which limits plasma total and unbound concentrations of methadone and prolongs the pharmacological actions of methadone in patients receiving a daily maintenance dose. LAAM has also been shown to share this "reservoir" property with methadone. Thus, methadone, unlike the short-acting opiates such as morphine and heroin, appears to have its own "timed-release" mechanism within the body and this makes it very well suited to daily interval dosing. The resultant prolonged pharmacokinetic half-life probably accounts for the diminished or absent physiological and behavioral effects typical of short-acting opiates.

(See Inturrisi, and Verebely, 1972; Sullivan et al., 1972; Dole and Kreek, 1973; Kreek, 1973d; Anggard et al., 1974; Hachey et al., 1977; Kreek et al., 1978; Kreek, Hachey, et al., 1979; Nakamura et al., 1982; Kreek, 1991c)

METHADONE MAINTENANCE

Treatment Regimen

In maintenance treatment of opiate addicts, methadone is administered as a single constant daily dose after the induction period is over. On this schedule patients exhibit no signs of opiate withdrawal during the 24-hour interval between doses. If a daily dose is missed or omitted, however, a patient on methadone maintenance will exhibit signs and symptoms of opiate withdrawal, usually within 24 to 36 hours after the last dose of methadone. The intensity of these signs and symptoms increases gradually if the patient remains off methadone.

A daily dose of methadone stabilizes a maintenance patient pharmacologically by the creation of a drug reservoir in the tissues of the body that holds the plasma level within narrow limits. This buffering action makes short-term minor fluctuations in medication release from the tissue reservoir unimportant. Although opiate withdrawal symptoms can be prevented with low doses, it is important to provide adequate treatment doses (60–120 mg/day in most patients) to assure plasma levels that "blockade" the effects of any superimposed short-acting opiates. The well-documented importance of constant, steady blood levels argues strongly against the sometimes-used practice of using methadone dose level as a reward or punishment variable in so-called "contingency contracting" or other behavioral interventions.

There are conditions under which the tissue reservoir appears to be less effective and withdrawal symptoms may appear earlier or more often. One of these is severe, chronic liver disease, such as postviral or alcoholic cirrhosis, which probably results in a reduction in the amount of hepatic storage capacity for methadone. Less severe liver disease does not seem to have this effect. Also, drug interactions of specific types may accelerate the metabolism of methadone and decrease its effectiveness (see below).

(See Dole et al., 1966; Kreek, 1973c; Kreek, 1978b; Kreek, Oratz, and Rothschild, 1978; Novick, Fanizza, et al., 1981; Kreek, 1983a; Novick, Kreek, Arns, et al., 1985; Ball and Ross, 1991, Kreek, 1991c.)

Effects, Side Effects, and Special Pharmacological Issues

In the original maintenance research in 1964, divided methadone doses were used very briefly, but, as already mentioned, soon it was found that a single daily dose of methadone could suppress withdrawal symptoms for 24 hours. Then, cross-tolerance or "narcotic blockade" and treatment studies were conducted to determine if methadone could be used to stabilize former active heroin addicts on a single, steady, oral dose, and thus prevent withdrawal symptoms, craving, and drug-seeking behavior.

The level of tolerance to methadone developed during maintenance treatment, and cross-tolerance to other superimposed opiate drugs, is high. In the 1964 research, the phenomenon of narcotic blockade was described in which cross-tolerance blocks the effect of any superimposed short-acting opiate drug. In double-blind studies conducted on former heroin addicts stabilized on full treatment doses of methadone, doses of heroin far exceeding those that might be used illicitly had no effects in the research subjects. Occasional medication errors have also been reported in which a stabilized, long-term, methadone-maintained patient has been given up to 10 times the usual dose of medication and, in most cases, there were no untoward effects except for somnolence.

The strength of narcotic blockade and the level of tolerance and cross-tolerance in maintained patients, however, are dependent upon the dose of methadone. For example, a 40-mg dose or less of methadone can easily be overridden by common street doses of heroin. Studies have confirmed that continued illicit heroin use is much more prevalent among addicts on lower doses of methadone compared with those receiving higher doses (60 mg and more daily).

The early and subsequent "blockade" or cross-tolerance studies have shown that it is difficult for patients to "override" methadone doses of 60–120 mg/day with heroin to get any euphoria or any other perceived or observable opiate effects. This lack of any override effect has been established in the clinical research laboratory and subsequently on the street. Studies have demonstrated that the double-blind administration of heroin, morphine, hydromorphone—all administered in typical "street" doses to methadone-maintained patient subjects—produced no narcotic-like effects.

In addition, single-blind administration of heroin in increasing doses to methadone-maintained research volunteers had no effects until the doses of heroin administered (up to 200 mg) exceeded street amounts commonly used at that time. Such studies have demonstrated that the margin of safety with respect to respiratory depression is very high. Consequently, if an individual maintained on methadone sought to get "high" on heroin (which frequently is attempted during the first few weeks in treatment), he or she is not likely to experience any desired or adverse effects.

Although some methadone is diverted to the street, the instances of primary addiction to methadone are extremely rare. Illicit methadone is used primarily by addicts to self-medicate for a short time for "detoxification" purposes or for extended periods in a "maintenance" mode. (See chapter 4 for an extended discussion of diversion.)

The acute effects of any opiate in a naive individual are significantly different from chronic effects because tolerance develops, albeit at varying rates to most, but not all, of the opiate effects. Diverse acute effects of opiates involving multiple organ systems have been recognized for years and more carefully defined and studied in recent years. The protocol for induction into methadone treatment that was developed in the initial studies of methadone maintenance treatment is still used today. During the first few weeks of maintenance treatment, the daily dose gradually is increased at a rate slow enough to prevent any appearance of narcotic-like effects.

From around two months onward, doses are held constant at an adequate "blockading" level, usually of 60 to 120 mg, to provide cross-tolerance and thus prevent any appearance of euphoria if the patient should attempt to superimpose the use of illicit heroin. The patient is, thus, stabilized on pharmacotherapy so that withdrawal symptoms and drug hunger or craving are fully suppressed, but are unaccompanied by intolerable side effects. The side effects, which may occur if methadone is used in doses exceeding the degree of tolerance developed, are somnolence, drowsiness, nausea, vomiting, insomnia, difficulty in urination, edema of the lower extremities, and constipation (to be discussed later). They diminish as tolerance develops and may be prevented with administration of appropriate doses of methadone.

Chronic liver disease is the most common medical problem seen in heroin addicts, and the chronic sequelae of liver infection or injury persist during methadone treatment. The majority of heroin addicts entering methadone maintenance treatment have biochemical evidence of chronic liver disease, and, until very recently, 80 to 90 percent have serological evidence of exposure to hepatitis B and/or hepatitis C. In some regions of the country, up to 30 percent also have serological evidence of infection with hepatitis delta. Of patients maintained on methadone for months to years, over one-half have persistent biochemical liver abnormalities. In these patients, the abnormalities result from the complications of previous heroin addiction and include viral hepatitis of one or more type, comorbidity with alcoholism, or both. Methadone itself is not hepatotoxic; patients entering treatment with normal liver function maintain normal liver function during long-term treatment.

Chronic renal disease is a medical problem in some heroin addicts entering methadone maintenance, but the presence of chronic renal disease does not result in the systemic accumulation of methadone or its metabolites. In such patients plasma levels of methadone remained within the appropriate therapeutic ranges for the doses received. This is because methadone metabolites are inactive; also, unlike morphine and heroin, methadone and its metabolites are normally excreted in part in feces as well as in urine and may be exclusively excreted by the hepatobiliary fecal route in the presence of renal disease.

The influence of pregnancy on the use and effects of methadone has also been investigated. Plasma concentrations of methadone are significantly lower and systemic elimination of methadone more rapid as pregnancy progresses through the third trimester. Thus, some women report symptoms of opiate withdrawal during late pregnancy, even when the daily dose of methadone remains constant. Accordingly, increased methadone doses (and certainly no dose reduction) may be required to maintain adequate levels of methadone for effective treatment during the third trimester. In addition to minimizing risk of relapse, it is important to suppress withdrawal symptoms, because they can trigger premature labor.

To date, the only adverse effects of methadone maintenance treatment on the fetus have been the production of physical dependence, which causes mild to modest opiate withdrawal signs and symptoms in the early postnatal period in many, but not all, babies. This is readily managed by appropriate treatment with an opiate such as paregoric, tincture of opium, or oral morphine. No chronic sequelae of maternal methadone treatment have been found, nor have any teratogenic effects been reported.

(See Dole et al., 1966; Cherubin et al., 1972; Gordon and Appel, 1972; Kreek, Dodesn, et al., 1972; Kreek, 1973a; Stimmel et al., 1973; Kreek, Schecter, Gutjahr, Bowen, et al., 1974; Kreek, 1978b; Kreek, 1979; Beverly et al., 1980; Kleber et al., 1980; Kreek, Gutjahr, and Hecht, 1980; Hartman et al., 1983; Kreek, 1983b; Novick, Farci, Karayiannis, 1985; Pond et al., 1985; Kreek, Khuri, et al., 1986; Novick, Khan, and Kreek, 1986; Novick, Stenger, et al., 1986; Kreek, Des Jarlais, et al., 1990; Kreek, 1991c; Kreek, 1992b; Novick, Richman, et al., 1993; Novick, Reagan, et al., in press.)

Physiological Functions Disrupted During Heroin Addiction

Addicts inject (or self-administer by another route) themselves repeatedly with increasingly larger doses of heroin, usually sufficient to achieve the desired euphoria or "high" effect during chronic use of opiates, and modified responses, or tolerance, to the drug develop. The first self-administrations of heroin by a curious adolescent are likely to cause nausea with or without an accompanying pleasurable feeling. Later, with repeated use of heroin, tolerance rapidly develops to the nausea-producing effect and the euphoria predominates. The euphoric experience becomes central to the addict's life; but with additional heroin use, the addict finds it progressively more difficult to achieve euphoria, unless an increasing dose of heroin is used.

Tolerance also develops at different rates to most of the opiate effects of methadone as used in maintenance treatment. Most of the initial opiate effects, predominantly somnolence, can be avoided by starting treatment at relatively low doses and increasing the dose gradually to appropriate treatment levels. Other important physiological functions that are deranged during cycles of heroin addiction include (1) central nervous system stress responses that are mediated by the hypothalamic-pituitary-adrenal axis; (2) reproductive biology hormones of the hypothalamic-pituitary gonadal axis with resultant abnormal function; (3) various indices of immune function that are linked to or modulated by neuroendocrine function. These altered functions, which may contribute to or be part of the mechanism underlying drug-seeking behavior, have been shown to normalize during long-term steady-dose methadone treatment.

Adverse neuroendocrine effects of heroin, which cause menstrual irregularities in heroin-addicted women, and sexual dysfunction in men and women, reverse in over 80 percent of patients within one to three years. Constipation, a side effect of both short- and long-acting opiates, persists for a protracted period of time; with slow development of tolerance, this effect on the gastrointestinal tract diminishes. Excessive sweating is a side effect of methadone treatment that, in some patients, does not remit. Some patients (less than 20 percent) continue to complain of sleep and sexual dysfunction for up to one year or longer, and may experience constipation for up to three years; up to 50 percent experience excessive sweating for even longer periods of time.

In contrast to the gradual development of tolerance expressed by reduction at different rates of these diverse side effects, tolerance to sedative and also analgesic effects of opiates develops rapidly and fully in methadone-maintained patients. Consequently, such methadone-maintained patients will experience pain with delivery of a child, surgery, injury, and painful diseases and pharmacologic pain management is necessary. Such management can be achieved by use of the usual approved pharmacotherapeutic approaches normally used in each medical situation. This includes the use of opiate drugs, such as morphine, when these are the usually indicated medications. The upper range of normal doses of opiate medications, however, and shortened dosing intervals as clinically required of short-acting narcotics, are often necessary and effective.

(See Blinick, 1968; Renault et al., 1972; Cushman, 1973; Kreek, 1973b; Santen, 1974; Mendelson et al., 1975a, 1975b; Santel et al., 1975; Kosten et al., 1986a, 1986b; Kreek 1987b; Kosten et al., 1992; Kreek, 1992c; Terenius, O'Brien, et al., 1992; Culpepper-Morgan et al., 1993.)

INTERACTIONS OF METHADONE WITH OTHER DRUGS

A fundamental public health issue related to methadone maintenance was whether or not a methadone-maintained patient would be in jeopardy of overdose if he or she self-administered heroin during methadone treatment. As noted above, the 1964 cross-tolerance studies documented that the risk of morbidity or death in methadone patients receiving a full treatment dose (60 to 120 mg per day) is extremely low because of the high level of tolerance (and cross-tolerance to other opiates) developed during treatment.

In addition to blocking the euphoric effects of superimposed, short-acting opiate drugs, methadone and its accompanying narcotic "blockade" may serve a relapse-prevention function. The suppression and ultimate "extinction" of drug-seeking behavior should result, theoretically at least, when illicit opiate self-administration is uncoupled from the anticipated and desired opiate effect of euphoria. The now well-documented significant reduction or cessation of illicit opiate use by former heroin addicts stabilized on steady and adequate doses of methadone suggests that this may be due partly to the effects of counseling, as well as to the direct biological effects of the drug.

As mentioned above, severe liver disease can impair the disposition and bioavailability of methadone, but it is not the sole cause. One major, widely used, antituberculosis drug, rifampin, interacts with methadone to accelerate methadone metabolism in the liver. This interaction is important because opiate addicts are particularly vulnerable to tuberculosis. Rifampin has been shown to alter significantly the clinical efficacy of methadone by accelerating its metabolism in the liver and thus its rapid removal from the body. This rapid biotransformation of methadone leads to the appearance of withdrawal symptoms in patients otherwise well-maintained on methadone. The two major effects of rifampin on methadone metabolism, a lowering of plasma concentrations and increased urinary excretion of the major metabolite, suggest that the drug exerts its effect by enhancing hepatic microsomal enzyme activity.

Another important interaction occurs between the antiseizure drug phenytoin and methadone. Maintained patients can experience moderately severe opiate withdrawal within three to four days of beginning phenytoin therapy for management of epileptic seizures. Studies have shown that phenytoin accelerates methadone metabolism, and methadone dosing adjustments need to be anticipated when phenytoin is initiated or discontinued.

Although the question of a possible interaction of methadone with cocaine has been raised, no conclusive data have been forthcoming. Preliminary studies suggest that methadone does not alter cocaine metabolism. However, some studies have suggested that cocaine may, in some cases, accelerate the metabolism of methadone.

Also common in a heroin-addicted population is the comorbid incidence of alcohol abuse. It is estimated that at least one in four or five heroin addicts, and former addicts maintained on methadone, abuse alcohol. Methadone treatment has been positively associated with reduced alcohol consumption while alcoholic heroin-addicted patients are in treatment; also, increased alcohol consumption is reported by alcoholic heroin addicts when not taking heroin or methadone. Disulfiram (Antabuse) has been used to deter alcoholic abusers from further drinking on the basis of aversive effects of the alcohol-disulfiram interaction. Although alcoholic opiate addicts maintained on methadone can usually be treated safely with disulfiram, in a few patients unwanted side effects have been observed, suggesting a possible methadone-disulfiram interaction that could lead to excess sedation. A theoretical basis for this effect could include a disulfiram-induced inhibition of the liver microsomal enzymes that are responsible for the metabolism of methadone, but such an interaction was not found in one study in which average doses of disulfiram were administered to methadone-maintained subjects. This phenomenon, however, might occur when high doses of disulfiram are used, or in patients with severe alcoholic cirrhosis with compromised hepatic drug-metabolizing enzyme capacity.

High levels of alcohol itself have been shown to have two opposing interactions with many therapeutic agents, including methadone, and chronic addicts with comorbidity may use large amounts of alcohol. Alcohol is metabolized by the hepatic microsomal enzymes. When present in large amounts, alcohol may retard the biotransformation of medications that are metabolized by the hepatic P450 enzyme related systems; yet when alcohol levels fall, drug metabolism may be accelerated due to the chronic effects of alcohol on hepatic microsomal enzyme activity.

(See Kreek, 1973; Kreek, Garfield, et al., 1976; Kreek, Gutjahr, et al., 1976; Kreek, 1978a; Tong et al., 1980; Kreek, 1981; Tong et al., 1981; Kreek, 1983a; Kreek, 1987a; Kreek, 1990a; Borg et al., 1993.)

IMPACT OF METHADONE MAINTENANCE ON INFECTIOUS DISEASES

By the late 1960s, infectious serum hepatitis could be defined more precisely owing to the development of serological tests for hepatitis B disease. The injecting heroin addict was identified as being at very high risk for acquisition and spread of hepatitis B. In multiple studies, over 80 percent of the injecting heroin addicts entering methadone treatment had markers of prior infection and 5 to 15 percent had hepatitis B antigenemia.[2] However, studies have also shown that after 10 years or more in maintenance treatment, the percentage of patients with hepatitis B antigenemia drops to less than 5 percent.

By the late 1970s a second and lethal form of hepatitis, caused by a viroid-like circular RNA agent (delta agent) that requires hepatitis B for its own infectiousness, was discovered and its biology defined. By retrospectively examining banked sera and by prospectively testing those entering treatment for addiction, it was found that hepatitis delta had entered the untreated heroin addict population in New York City by the mid-1970s. By 1984, approximately 90 percent of the untreated heroin addicts on the streets of New York City

---

[2] A positive marker for hepatitis B virus antigen, indicating the presence of live hepatitis B virus and thus potential viral replication.

continued to show evidence of having been infected with hepatitis B, as evidenced by the presence of some marker for that disease; and approximately 30 percent by that time had evidence of hepatitis delta infection. Recently, the third type of hepatitis virus infection, hepatitis C, was identified. Studies have shown hepatitis C virus infection in 80 to 90 percent of heroin addicts and former heroin addicts in methadone treatment.

In 1981, shortly after the clinical symptoms of AIDS were characterized, the etiological viral agent HIV-1 was identified. By examining blood samples that had been banked prospectively from 1969 onward, it was found that HIV-1 infection had reached the drug-injecting population in New York City in 1978 and infection had progressed rapidly until 1983–1984, when the prevalence of HIV-1 infection reached a level of over 50 percent of intravenous users in the inner city area. Of public health importance, investigators further found that heroin addicts in New York City who had entered effective methadone maintenance treatment programs before the 1978 advent of the AIDS epidemic and who remained in treatment displayed a much lower incidence of HIV-1 infection in 1984 than did untreated heroin addicts: less than 10 percent of such methadone patients were infected in 1984, compared to over 50 percent of untreated heroin addicts. Studies of HIV-1 infection in long-term, methadone-maintained patients have been reported in Sweden and other countries worldwide with similar findings of efficacy of methadone treatment in the prevention of HIV-1 infection.

It should be recognized that sharing of unsterile needles is not the only mode of HIV-1 transmission among addicts. Cocaine use by methadone patients is also a risk factor for HIV-1 infection, owing to promiscuous sexual behavior commonly associated with cocaine, including sex as payment for the drug. Concurrent use of cocaine by heroin addicts is estimated to be between 50 and 90 percent and, thus, is an added risk factor in the heroin-using population. Once in treatment, the prevalence of cocaine use among heroin addicts generally drops to between 20 and 40 percent.

Finally, and of potentially great importance, studies have shown that multiple indices of immune function are deranged during cycles of heroin addiction, probably because of many factors, including lifestyle, multiple infectious diseases, and possible direct or indirect effects of the drug use. Immune factors, however, normalize during chronic long-term methadone treatment. Natural killer cell activity is not altered by methadone *in vitro*. Long-term methadone maintenance permits return to normal levels of natural killer cell activity, as well as to normal absolute numbers of B cells and T cell subsets, which may have important implications for immune system function and, possibly, for retarding the progress of HIV-1 infection to AIDS.

(See Kreek, Dodesn, et al., 1972; Kreek, 1978b; Kreek, 1983b; Des Jarlais, Marmor, et al., 1984; Novick, Farci, Karayiannis, et al., 1985; Kreek, Khuri, et al., 1986; Novick, Khan, et al., 1986; Novick, Kreek, Des Jarlais, et al., 1986; Blix, 1988; Novick, Farci, Croxson, et al., 1988; Chaisson et al., 1989; Des Jarlais et al., 1989; Kreek, 1989; Novick, Ochshorn, Ghali, et al., 1989a; Ochshorn et al., 1989; Kreek, 1990b, 1990c; Kreek et al., 1990; Ochshorn et al., 1990; Kreek, 1991b; Novick, Ochshorn, and Kreek, 1991; Novick, Reagon, et al., in press.)

REFERENCES

Albeck, H, Woodfield, S, and Kreek, MJ. 1989. Quantitative and pharmacokinetic analysis of naloxone in plasma using high performance liquid chromatography with electrochemical detection and solid phase extraction. *Journal of Chromatography* 488:435–445.

Anggard, E, Gunne, L-M, Holmstrand, J, McMahon, RE, Sandberg, C-G, and Sullivan, HR. 1974. Disposition of methadone in methadone maintenance. *Clinical Pharmacology and Therapeutics* 17(3):258–266.

Ball, JC, and Ross, A. 1991. *The Effectiveness of Methadone Maintenance Treatment: Patients, Programs, Services and Outcome.* New York: Springer-Verlag.

Beverly, CL, Kreek, MJ, Wells, AO, and Curtis, JL. 1980. Effects of alcohol abuse on progression of liver disease in methadone-maintained patients. In: *Problems of Drug Dependence, 1979; Proceedings of the 41st Annual Scientific Meeting of the Committee on Problems of Drug Dependence*, L.S. Harris, ed., NIDA Research Monograph 27 Series., Rockville, Md., Pp. 399-401.

Blinick, G. 1968. Menstrual function and pregnancy in narcotics addicts treated with methadone. *Nature* 219:180.

Blix, O. 1988. AIDS and IV heroin addicts: The preventive effect of methadone maintenance in Sweden. *Proceedings of the 4th International Conference on AIDS, Stockholm.*

Borg, L, Ho, A, and Kreek, MJ. 1993. Availability of reliable serum methadone determination for management of symptomatic patients. In: *Problems of Drug Dependence, 1992; Proceedings of the 54th Annual Scientific Meeting of the College on Problems of Drug Dependence.* L.S. Harris, ed. National Institute on Drug Abuse Research Monograph 132, Rockville, Md., DHHS Publication No. (ADM) 93-3505. P. 221.

Branch, AD, Benefeld, BJ, Baroudy, BM, Wells, FV, Gerin, JL, and Robertson, HD. 1989. A UV-sensitive RNA structural element in a viroid-like domain of the hepatitis delta virus. *Science* 243:649–652.

Branch, AD, Unterwald, EM, Lee, SE, and Kreek, MJ. 1992. Quantitation of preproenkephalin mRNA levels in brain regions from male Fischer rats following chronic cocaine treatment using a recently developed solution hybridization procedure. *Molecular Brain Research* 14:231–238.

Chaisson, RE, Bacchetti, P, Osmond, D, Brodie, B, Sande, MA, and Moss, AR. 1989. Cocaine use and HIV infection in intravenous drug users in San Francisco. *Journal of the American Medical Association* 261:561–565.

Chen, Y, Mestek, A, Liu, J, Hurley, JA, and Yu, L. 1993a. Molecular cloning and functional expression of a mu opioid receptor from rat brain. *Molecular Pharmacology* 44:8–12.

Chen, Y, Mestek, A, Liu, J, and Yu, L. 1993b. Molecular cloning of a rat kappa opioid receptor reveals sequence similarities to the mu and delta opioid receptors. *Biochemical Journal* 295:625–628.

Cherubin, CE, Kane, S, Weinberger, DR, et al. 1972. Persistence of transaminase abnormalities in former drug addicts. *Annals of Internal Medicine* 76:385.

Culpepper-Morgan, JA, Inturrisi, CE, Portenoy, RK, Foley, K, Houde, RW, Marsh, F, and Kreek, MJ. 1993. Treatment of opioid induced constipation with oral naloxone: A pilot study. *Clinical Pharmacology and Therapeutics* 23:90–95.

Cushman, P, Jr. 1973. Plasma testosterone in narcotic addiction. *American Journal of Medicine* 55:452–458.

Des Jarlais, DC, Friedman, SR, Novick, DM, Sotheran, JL, Thomas, P, Yancovitz, SR, Mildvan, D, Weber, J, Kreek, MJ, Maslansky, R, Bartelme, S, Spira, T, and Marmor, M. 1989. HIV I infection among intravenous drug users in Manhattan, New York City 1977 to 1987. *Journal of the American Medical Association* 261:1008–1012.

Des Jarlais, DC, Marmor, M, Cohen, H, Yancovitz, S, Garber, J, Friedman, S, Kreek, MJ, Miescher, A, Khuri, E, Friedman, SM, Rothenberg, R, Echenberg, D, O'Malley, PO, Braff, E, Chin, J, Burtenol, P and Sikes, RK. 1984. Antibodies to a retrovirus etiologically associated with Acquired Immuno-deficiency Syndrome (AIDS) in populations with increased incidences of the syndrome. *Morbidity and Mortality Weekly Report* 33:377–379.

Dole, VP. 1970. Biochemistry of addiction. *Annual Review of Biochemistry* 39:821–240.

Dole, VP. 1988. Implications of methadone maintenance for theories of narcotic addiction. *Journal of the American Medical Association* 260:3025–3029.

Dole, VP, and Kreek, MJ. 1973. Methadone plasma level: Sustained by a reservoir of drug in tissue. *Proceedings of the National Academy of Sciences* 70:10.

Dole, VP, Nyswander, ME, and Kreek, MJ. 1966. Narcotic blockade. *Archives of Internal Medicine* 118:304–309.

Evans, CJ, Keith, DE, Jr., Morrison, H, Magendzo, K, Edwards, RH. 1992. Cloning of a delta opioid receptor by functional expression. *Science* 258:1952–1955.

Goldstein, A, Lowney, LT, and Pal, BK. 1971. Stereospecific and nonspecific interactions of the morphine congener levorphanol in subcellular fractions of mouse brain. *Proceedings of the National Academy of Sciences of the United States of America* 68:1742–1747.

Goldstein, A, and Freeman, WH. 1994. *Addiction: From Biology to Drug Policy*, New York.

Gordon, NB, and Appel, PW. 1972. Performance of effectiveness in relation to methadone maintenance. In: *National Association for the Prevention of Addiction to Narcotics, Proceedings of the Fourth National Conference on Methadone Treatment*. Pp. 425–427.

Hachey, DL, Kreek, MJ and Mattson, DH. 1977. Quantitative analysis of methadone in biological fluids using deuterium-labeled methadone and GLC-chemical-ionization mass spectrometry. *Journal of Pharmaceutical Sciences* 66:1579–1582.

Hartman, N, Kreek, MJ, Ross, A, Khuri, E, Millman, RB, and Rodriguez, R. 1983. Alcohol use in youthful methadone maintained former heroin addicts: Liver impairment and treatment outcome. *Alcoholism, Clinical, and Experimental Research* 7:316–320.

Hughes, J, Smith, TW, Kosterlitz, HW, Fothergill, LA, Morgan, BA, and Morris, HR. 1975. Identification of two related pentapeptides from the brain with potent opiate agonist activity. *Nature* 258:577–580.

Hurd, YL, Brown, EE, Finlay, JM, Fibiger, HC, and Gerfen, CR. 1992. Cocaine self-administration differentially alters mRNA expression of striatal peptides. *Molecular Brain Research* 13:165–170.

Ingoglia, NA, and Dole, VP. 1970. Localization of d- and l-methadone after intra ventricular injection into rat brain. *Journal of Pharmacology and Therapeutics* 175:84–87.

Inturrisi, CE, and Verebely, K. 1972. The levels of methadone in the plasma in methadone maintenance. *Clinical Pharmacology and Therapeutics* 13:633–637.

Kieffer, BL, Befort, K, Gaveriaux-Ruff, C, and Hirth, CG. 1992. The delta-opioid receptor: Isolation of a cDNA by expression cloning and pharmacological characterization. *Proceedings of the National Academy of Sciences* 89:12,048–12,052.

Kleber, HD, Slobetz, F, and Mezritz, M, eds. 1980. *Medical Evaluation of Long-Term Methadone-Maintained Clients.* National Institute on Drug Abuse. DHHS Publication No. (ADM) 81-1029. Washington, D.C.: U.S. Government Printing Office.

Kosten, TR, Kreek, MJ, Raghunath, J, and Kleber, HD. 1986a. Cortisol levels during chronic naltrexone maintenance treatment in ex-opiate addicts. *Biological Psychiatry* 21:217–220.

Kosten, TR, Kreek, MJ, Raghunath, J, and Kleber, HD. 1986b. A preliminary study of beta-endorphin during chronic naltrexone maintenance treatment in ex-opiate addicts. *Life Sciences* 39: 55–59.

Kosten, TR, Morgan, C, and Kreek, MJ. 1992. Beta-endorphin levels during heroin, methadone, buprenorphine and naloxone challenges: Preliminary findings. *Biological Psychology* 32:523–528.

Kreek, MJ. 1973a. Medical safety and side effects of methadone in tolerant individuals. *Journal of the American Medical Association* 223:665–668.

Kreek, MJ. 1973b. Physiological implications of methadone treatment. In: *Methadone Treatment Manual.* U.S. Department of Justice. Publication No. 2700-00227. Washington, D.C.: U.S. Government Printing Office. Pp. 85–91.

Kreek, MJ. 1973c. Physiological implications of methadone treatment. In: National Association for the Prevention of Addiction to Narcotics, *Proceedings of the Fifth National Conference on Methadone Treatment.* Pp. 85–91.

Kreek, MJ. 1973d. Plasma and urine levels of methadone. *New York State Journal of Medicine* 73:2773–2777.

Kreek, MJ. 1978a. Effects of drugs and alcohol on opiate disposition and action. In: *Factors Affecting the Action of Narcotics*, M.W. Adler, L. Manara, and R Samnin, eds. New York: Raven Press. Pp. 717–739a.

Kreek, MJ. 1978b. Medical complications in methadone patients. *Annals of the New York Academy of Sciences* 311:110–134.

Kreek, MJ. 1979. Methadone disposition during the perinatal period in humans. *Pharmacology Biochemistry Behavior.* 11(Suppl.):1–7.

Kreek, MJ. 1981. Metabolic interactions between opiates and alcohol. *Annals of the New York Academy of Sciences* 362:36–49.

Kreek, MJ. 1983a. Factors modifying the pharmacological effectiveness of methadone. In: *Research in the Treatment of Narcotic Addiction: State of the Art,* J.R. Cooper, F. Altman, B.S. Brown, and D. Czechowicz, eds. NIDA Research Monograph Series, Rockville, Md., DHHS Publication No. (ADM) 83-1281. Pp. 95–114a.

Kreek, MJ. 1983b. Health consequences associated with use of methadone. In: *Research in the Treatment of Narcotic Addiction: State of the Art,* J.R. Cooper, F. Altman, B.S. Brown, and D. Czechowicz, eds. NIDA Monograph Series, Rockville, Md., DHHS Publication No. (ADM) 83-1281. Pp. 456–482.

Kreek, MJ. 1987a. Multiple drug abuse patterns and medical consequences. In: *Psychopharmacology: The Third Generation of Progress,* H.Y. Meltzer, ed. New York: Raven Press. Pp. 1597–1604.

Kreek, MJ. 1987b. Tolerance and dependence: Implications for the pharmacological treatment of addiction. In: *Problems of Drug Dependence, 1986; Proceedings of the 48th Annual Scientific Meeting of The Committee on Problems of Drug Dependence,* L.S. Harris, ed. NIDA Research Monograph Series, Rockville, Md., DHHS Publication No.(ADM) 87-1508. Pp. 76:53–61.

Kreek, MJ. 1989. Immunological approaches to clinical issues in drug abuse. In: *Problems of Drug Dependence, 1988; Proceedings of the 50th Annual Scientific Meeting of the Committee on Problems of Drug Dependence.* L.S. Harris, ed. NIDA Research Monograph 90, Rockville, Md., DHHS Publication No. (ADM) 89-1605. Pp. 77–86, 1989.

Kreek, MJ. 1990a. Drug interactions in humans related to drug abuse and its treatment. *Modern Methods in Pharmacology* 6:265–282.

Kreek, MJ. 1990b. HIV infection and parenteral drug abuse: Ethical issues in diagnosis, treatment, research and the maintenance of confidentiality. In: *Proceedings of the Third International Congress on Ethics in Medicine*—Nobel Conference Series. P. Allebeck and B. Jansson, eds. New York: Raven Press. Pp. 181–188.

Kreek, MJ. 1990c. Immune function in heroin addicts and former heroin addicts in treatment: Pre/post AIDS epidemic. *Current Chemical and Pharmacological Advances on Drugs of Abuse Which Alter Immune Function and Their Impact Upon HIV Infection,* P.T.K. Pham and K. Rice, eds. NIDA Research Monograph 96, Rockville, Md. Pp. 192–219.

Kreek, MJ. 1991b. Immunological function in active heroin addicts and methadone maintained former addicts: Observations and possible mechanisms. In: *Problems of Drug Dependence, 1990; Proceedings of the 52nd Annual Scientific Meeting of the Committee on Problems of Drug Dependence.* L.S. Harris, ed. NIDA Research Monograph 105, Rockville, Md., DHHS Publication No. (ADM) 91-1753. Pp. 75–81.

Kreek, MJ. 1991c. Using methadone effectively: Achieving goals by application of laboratory, clinical, and evaluation research and by development of innovative programs. In: *Improving Drug Abuse Treatment*, R. Pickens, C. Leukefeld, and C.R. Schuster, eds. NIDA Research Monograph106. Rockville, Md. Pp. 245–266.

Kreek, MJ. 1992a. The addict as a patient. In: *Substance Abuse: A Comprehensive Textbook*, J.H. Lowinson, P. Ruiz, R.B. Millman, and J.G. Langrod, eds. Baltimore: Williams & Wilkins. Pp. 997–100.

Kreek, MJ. 1992b. Epilogue: Medical maintenance treatment for heroin addiction, from a retrospective and prospective viewpoint. In: *State Methadone Maintenance Treatment Guidelines*. Office for Treatment Improvement, Division for State Assistance. Pp. 255–272. November.

Kreek, MJ. 1992c. Rationale for maintenance pharmacotherapy of opiate dependence. In: *Addictive States*, C.P. O'Brien and J.H. Jaffe, eds. New York: Raven Press. Pp. 205–230.

Kreek, MJ, Des Jarlais, DC, Trepo, CL, Novick, DM, Abdul-Quader, A, and Raghunath, J. 1990. Contrasting prevalence of delta hepatitis markers in parenteral drug abusers with and without AIDS. *Journal of Infectious Diseases* 162:538–541.

Kreek, MJ, Dodes, L, Kane, S, Knobler, J, and Martin, R. 1972. Long-term methadone maintenance therapy: Effects on liver function. *Annals of Internal Medicine* 77:598–602.

Kreek, MJ, Garfield, JW, Gutjahr, CL, and Giusti, LM. 1976. Rifampin-induced methadone withdrawal. *New England Jouranl of Medicine* 294:1104–1106.

Kreek, MJ, Gutjahr, CL, Garfield, JW, Bowen, DV and Field, FH. 1976. Drug interactions with methadone. *Annals of the New York Academy of Sciences* 281:350–370.

Kreek, MJ, Hachey, DL, and Klein, PD. 1979. Stereoselective disposition of methadone in man. *Life Sciences* 24:925–932.

Kreek, MJ, and Hartman, N. 1982. Chronic use of opioids and antipsychotic drugs: Side effects, effects on endogenous opioids and toxicity. *Annals of the New York Academy of Sciences* 398:151–172.

Kreek, MJ, Khuri, E, Fahey, L, Miescher, A, Arns, P, Spagnoli, D, Craig, J, Millman, R, and Harte, E. 1986. Long term follow-up studies of the medical status of adolescent former heroin addicts in chronic methadone maintenance treatment: Liver disease and immune status. In: *Problems of Drug Dependence, 1985; Proceedings of the 47th Annual Scientific Meeting of The Committee on Problem of Drug Dependence*. L.S. Harris, ed. NIDA Research Monograph 67, Rockville, Md., DHHS Publication No.(ADM) 86-1448. Pp. 307–309.

Kreek, MJ, Oratz, M, and Rothschild, MA. 1978. Hepatic extraction of long-and short-acting narcotics in the isolated perfused rabbit liver. *Gastroenterology* 75:88–94.

Kreek, MJ, Raghunath, J, Plevy, S, Hamer, D, Schneider, B, and Hartman, N. 1984 ACTH, cortisol and beta-endorphin response to metyrapone testing during chronic methadone maintenance treatment in humans. *Neuropeptides* 5:277–278. Kreek, MJ, Schaefer, RA, Hahn, EF, and Fishman, J. 1983. Naloxone, a specific opioid antagonist, reverses chronic idiopathic constipation. *Lancet* (Feb. 5) 261–262.

Kreek, MJ, Schecter, A, Gutjahr, CL, Bowen, D, Field, F, Queenan, J, and Merkatz, I. 1974. Analyses of methadone and other drugs in maternal and neonatal body fluids: Use in evaluation of symptoms in a neonate of mother maintained on methadone. *American Journal of Drug and Alcohol Abuse* 1:409–419.

Kreek, MJ, Schecter, AJ, Gutjahr, CL, and Hecht, M. 1980. Methadone use in patients with chronic renal disease. *Drug and Alcohol Dependence* 5:197–205.

Kreek, MJ, Schneider, BS, Raghunath, J, and Plevy, S. 1984. Prolonged (24 hour) infusion of the opioid antagonist naloxone does not significantly alter plasma levels of cortisol and ACTH in humans. *Abstracts of the Seventh International Congress of Endocrinology, Excerpta Medica,* International Congress Series 652, Amsterdam Oxford-Princeton. P. 845. July.

Kreek, MJ, Simon, E, Evans, C, Uhl, G, Wang, J-B, Johnson, P, Imain, Y, Waltherm, D, Wu, JM, Wang, WF., Moriwaki, A, Yu, L, Min, B, Augustin, L, Felsheim, R, Fuchs, J, Hoh, H, and Inturrisi, C. In press. Symposium for 20th anniversary. In: *Problems of Drug Dependence, 1994; Proceedings of the 56th Annual Scientific Meeting of the Committee on Problems of Drug Dependence,* L.S. Harris, ed. NIDA Research Monograph Series, Rockville, Md.

Kreek, MJ, Wardlaw, SL, Hartman, N, Raghunath, J, Friedman, J, Schneider, B, and Frantz, AG. 1983. Circadian rhythms and levels of beta-endorphin, ACTH, and cortisol during chronic methadone maintenance treatment in humans. *Life Sciences* 33 (Suppl. I):409–411.

McGinty, JF, Daunais, JB, and Roberts, CS. 1993. Cocaine self-administration causes an increase in preprodynorphin, but not c-fos, mRNA in rat Striatum. In: Problems of Drug Dependence, 1992: Proceedings of the 54th Annual Scientific Meeting of the Committee on Problems of Drug Dependence, NIDA Research Monograph Series, Rockville, Md. P. 143.

Mendelson, JH, Mendelson, JE, and Patch, YD. 1975a. Plasma testosterone levels in heroin addiction and during methadone maintenance. *Journal of Pharmacology and Experimental Therapeutics* 192:211–217.

Mendelson, JH, Meyer, RE, Ellingboe, J, et al. 1975b. Effects of heroin and methadone on plasma cortisol and testosterone. *Journal of Pharmacology and Experimental Therapeutics* 195:296–302.

Nakamura, K, Hachey, DL, Kreek, MJ, Irving, CS, and Klein, PD. 1982. Quantitation of methadone enantiomers in humans using stable isotope-labeled $^2H_3$, $^2H_5$, $^2H_8$ methadone. *Journal of Pharmaceutical Sciences* 71:39–43.

Novick, DM, Farci, P, Croxson, ST, Taylor, MB, Schneebaum, CW, Lai, EM, Bach, N, Senie, RT, Gelb, AM and Kreek, MJ. 1988. Hepatitis delta virus and human immunodeficiency virus antibodies in parenteral drug abusers who are hepatitis B surface antigen positive. *Journal of Infectious Diseases* 158:795–803.

Novick, DM, Farci, P, Karayiannis, P, Gelb, AM, Stenger, RJ, Kreek, MJ, and Thomas, HC. 1985. Hepatitis D virus antibody in HBsAg-positive and HBsAg-negative substance abusers with chronic liver disease. *Journal of Medical Virology* 15:351–356.

Novick, DM, Khan, I, and Kreek, MJ. 1986. Acquired immunodeficiency syndrome and infection with hepatitis viruses in individuals abusing drugs by injection. *United Nations Bulletin on Narcotics* 38:15–25.

Novick, DM, Kreek, MJ, Arns, PA, Lau, LL, Yancovitz, SR, and Gelb, AM. 1985. Effects of severe alcoholic liver disease on the disposition of methadone in maintenance patients. *Alcoholism, Clinical and Experimental Research* 9:349– 354.

Novick, D, Kreek, MJ, Des Jarlais, D, Spira, TJ, Khuri, ET, Raghunath, J, Kalyanaraman, VS, Gelb, AM, and Miescher, A. 1986. Antibody to LAV, the putative agent of AIDS, in parenteral drug abusers and methadone-maintained patients: Abstract of clinical research findings: Therapeutic, historical, and ethical aspects. In: *Problems of Drug Dependence, 1985; Proceedings of the 47th Annual Scientific Meeting of the Committee on Problems of Drug Dependence.* L.S. Harris, ed. NIDA Research Monograph Series, Rockville, Md., DHHS Publication No. (ADM) 86-1448. Pp. 318–320.

Novick, DM, Kreek, MJ, Fanizza, AM, Yancovitz, SR, Gelb, AM, and Stenger, RJ. 1981. Methadone disposition in patients with chronic liver disease. *Clinical Pharmacology and Therapeutics* 30:353–362.

Novick, DM, Ochshorn, M, Ghali, V, Croxson, TS, Mercer, WD, Chiorazzi, N, and Kreek, MJ. 1989. Natural killer cell activity and lymphocyte subsets in parenteral heroin abusers and long-term methadone maintenance patients. *Journal of Pharmacology and Experimental Therapeutics* 250:606–610.

Novick, DM, Ochshorn, M, and Kreek, MJ. 1991. In vivo and in vitro studies of opiates and cellular immunity in narcotic addicts. In: *Drugs of Abuse, Immunity and Immunodeficiency,* H. Friedman, In press. New York: Plenum Press. Pp. 159–170.

Novick, DM, Reagan, KJ, Croxson, TS, Gelb, AM, Stenger, RJ, and Kreek, MJ. Hepatitis C virus serology in parenteral drug users with chronic liver disease. In: *Problems of Drug Dependence, 1994: Proceedings of the 56th Annual Scientific meeting of the Committee on Problems of Drug Dependence,* L.S. Harris, ed. NIDA Research Monograph Series, Rockville, Md.

Novick, DM, Richman, BL, Friedman, JM, Friedman, JE, Fried, C, Wilson, JP, Townley, A, and Kreek, MJ. 1993. The medical status of methadone maintained patients in treatment for 11–18 years. *Drug and Alcohol Dependence* 33:235–245.

Novick, DM, Stenger, RJ, Gelb, AM, Most, J, Yancovitz, SR, and Kreek, MJ. 1986. Chronic liver disease in abusers of alcohol and parenteral drugs: A report of 204 consecutive biopsy-proven cases. *Alcoholism, Clinical, and Experimental Research* 10:500–505.

Ochshorn, M, Kreek, MJ, Khuri, E, Fahey, L, Craig, J, Aldana, MC, and Albeck, H. 1989. Normal and abnormal natural killer (NK) activity in methadone maintenance treatment patients. In: *Problems of Drug Dependence, 1988; Proceedings of the 50th Annual Scientific Meeting of the Committee on Problems of Drug Dependence,* L.S. Harris, ed. NIDA Research Monograph Series, Rockville, Md., DHHS Publication No. (ADM) 89-1605. P. 369.

Ochshorn, M, Novick, DM, and Kreek, MJ. 1990. In vitro studies of methadone effect on natural killer (NK) cell activity. *Israel Journal of Medical Sciences* 26:421–425.

Pert, CB, and Snyder, SH. 1973. Opiate receptor: demonstration in nervous tissue. *Science* 179:1011–1014.

Pescor, MJ. 1943. Follow-up study of treated narcotic drug addicts. *Public Health Report* (Suppl.)170:1.

Pond, SM, Kreek, MJ, Tong, TG, Raghunath, J, and Benowitz, NL. 1985. Altered methadone pharmacokinetics in methadone-maintained pregnant women. *Journal of Pharmacology and Experimental Therapeutics* 233:1–6.

Renault, PF, Schuster, CR, Heinrich, RL, et al. 1972. Altered plasma cortisol response in patients on methadone maintenance. *Clinical Pharmacology and Therapeutics* 13:269–273.

Santen, RJ. 1974. How narcotics addiction affects reproductive function in women. *Contemporary OB/GYN* 3:93–95.

Santen, RJ, Sofsky, J, Bilic, N, et al. 1975. Mechanism of action of narcotics in the production of menstrual dysfunction in women. *Fertility and Sterility* 26:538–548.

Simon, EJ, Hiller, JM, and Edelman, I. 1973. Stereospecific binding of the potent narcotic analgesic [3H]Etorphine to rat-brain homogenate. *Proceedings of the National Academy of Sciences* 70:1947–1949.

Spangler, R, Unterwald, EM, Branch, A, Ho, A, and Kreek, MJ. 1993a. Chronic cocaine administration increases prodynorphin mRNA levels in the caudate putamen of rats. In: *Problems of Drug Dependence, 1992; Proceedings of the 54th Annual Scientific Meeting of the Committee on Problems of Drug Dependence.* L.S. Harris, ed, NIDA Research Monograph Series, Rockville, Md. DHHS Publication No. (ADM) 93-3505. P. 142.

Spangler, R, Unterwald, EM, and Kreek, MJ. 1993b. "Binge" cocaine administration induces a sustained increase of prodynorphin mRNA in rat caudate-putamen. *Molecular Brain Research* 19:323–327.

Spangler, R, Zhou, Y, Unterwald, EM, and Kreek, MJ. In press. Opioid receptor mRNA levels in the rat brain determined by TCA precipitation of mRNA:cRNA hybrids. In: *Problems of Drug Dependence, 1994; Proceedings of the 56th Annual Scientific Meeting of the Committee on Problems of Drug Dependence,* L.S. Harris, ed. NIDA Research Monograph Series, Rockville, Md.

Stimmel, B, Vernace, S, Heller, E, et al. 1973. Hepatitis B antigen and antibody in former heroin addicts on methadone maintenance: Correlation with clinical and histological findings. In: *National Association for the Prevention of Addiction to Narcotics, Proceedings of the Fifth National Conference on Methadone Treatment.* Vol. 1. New York: NAPAN. Pp. 501–513.

Sullivan, HR, Smits, SE, Due, SL, Booher, RE, and McMahon, RE. 1972. Metabolism of *d*-methadone: Isolation and identification of analgesically active metabolites. *Life Sciences* 11(1):1093–1104.

Terenius, L. 1973. Stereospecific interaction between narcotic analgesics and a synaptic plasma membrane fraction of rat cerebral cortex. *Acta Pharmacologica ET Toxicologica* 32:317–320.

Terenius, L, and O'Brien, CP. 1992. Receptors and endogenous ligands: Implications for addiction. In: *Addictive States* CP O'Brien and JH Jaffe, eds. New York: Raven Press. Pp. 123-130.

Tong, TG, Benowitz, NL, and Kreek, MJ. 1980. Methadone-disulfiram interaction during methadone maintenance. *Journal of Clinical Pharmacology* 20:506–513.

Tong, TG, Pond, SM, Kreek, MJ, Jaffery, NF, and Benowitz, NL. 1981. Phenytoin-induced methadone withdrawal. *Annals of Internal Medicine* 94:349–351.

Unterwald, EM, Horne-King, J, and Kreek, MJ. 1993. Chronic cocaine alters brain mu opioid receptors. *Brain Research* 584:314–318.

Unterwald, EM, Rubenfeld, JM, Spangler, R, Wang, JB, Uhl, GR, and Kreek, MJ. 1994. Mu opioid receptor mRNA levels following chronic naltrexone administration. *Abstracts of the International Narcotics Research Conference.*

Unterwald, EM, Rubenfeld, JM, and Kreek, MJ. In press. Repeated cocaine administration upregulates κ and μ, but not δ, opioid receptors. *NeuroReport.*

Wang, JB, Imai, Y, Eppler, CM, Gregor, P, Spivak, C, and Uhl, GR. 1993. Mu-opiate receptor: cDNA cloning and expression. *Proceedings of the National Academy of Sciences* 90:10,230–10,234.

Yasuda, K, Raynor, K, Kong, H, Breder, CD, Takeda, J, Reisine, T, and Bell, GI. 1993. Cloning and functional comparison of kappa and delta opioid receptors from mouse brain. *Proceedings of the National Academy of Sciences* 90:6736–6740.

3

Who Are the Recipients of Treatment?

Policymakers and the interested public have a number of questions about heroin use and addiction. These questions include the following. How large is the population of heroin users and addicts? Does it appear to be growing or shrinking? How are heroin addicts distributed geographically and demographically in the population? What other substances do heroin addicts use that are detrimental to their well-being? What concurrent medical and social problems do heroin addicts have for which they need services? How persistent is heroin addiction if untreated? How likely are heroin addicts to seek treatment? What are the characteristics of those who do and do not seek treatment?

The major sources of information about the frequency of heroin use and addiction are general and special population surveys and information obtained from persons arrested for possession or sale of illegal drugs and those in treatment. Each data source has its limitations and no single source provides all the information that might be desired. Consequently, following this introductory discussion this chapter discusses respectively, data from population-oriented, addict-oriented, and treatment-oriented information sources.

The limitations of data about illicit substance abuse are intertwined with issues of concept and definition. There is no official psychiatric diagnosis termed "opiate addiction," the disorder that methadone programs treat. Instead, the newly published DSM-IV offers the following diagnoses: opiate dependence, opiate abuse, opiate intoxication, opiate withdrawal. Dependence requires three or more of the following symptoms occurring within a 12-month period: tolerance; withdrawal; taking larger amounts or taking amounts over a longer period than was intended; persistent desire or failed efforts to reduce or control use of the substance; spending a great deal of time obtaining the substance, using it, or recovering from its use; giving up important social, occupational, or recreational activities because of substance use; and continued use despite knowledge of a persistent physical or psychological problem likely to have been caused by use of the substance.

Addiction, as defined by Dorland's Medical Dictionary, would fall within the dependence diagnosis, but would be somewhat more severe. It requires, in addition to regular heavy use, four symptoms. One of these is dependence (physical or psychological); the others are a tendency to increase dosage (which is equivalent to tolerance in the dependence diagnosis), an overwhelming desire or need (compulsion) to continue use and to obtain the drug by any means (which appears in the DSM-IV definition of dependence as use in larger amounts than intended and inability to stop use, even when the drug's detrimental effects are known), and a detrimental effect on the individual and society (which appears in the DSM-IV definition of dependence as giving up social, recreational, and occupational activities to use the drug).

In addition to these efforts to definition the states experienced by individuals (e.g., tolerance, dependence, addiction) there are also various descriptions of a continuum regarding the use or consumption of drugs, legal and illicit. These descriptions include (1) "occasional use to regular use" (CDC, 1987), (2) "use, abuse, dependence, and recovery" (Gerstein and Harwood, 1990), and (3) "general use versus problematic use" (Reuter, 1993). For the purposes of this chapter, we will adopt a similar approach to analyzing the data. Specifically, we will discuss the continuum of those who ever used opiates, those who ever become dependent on opiates, those who become addicted, and those addicts who have been treated.

The data, drawn from multiple sources, show a steady reduction in numbers along this continuum. The vast majority of Americans have never used a self-administered, nonprescribed opiate. Of those who have used one, about half do not proceed beyond occasional use. Others progress to a relatively brief period of dependence (Biernackie, 1986) and cease use without treatment.

At the other end of the continuum, however, are those who engage in substantial use over long periods, become dependent, and fail at voluntarily ending their dependence. These are the addicts for whom methadone treatment is intended, treatment that has given rise to the methadone regulations. Although they represent a relatively small percentage of the total users of opiates, addicts constitute a large absolute number who contribute disportionately to drug-related crime and threats to the public health. Much more is known about the heroin addict group than about those who use heroin occasionally or are briefly dependent on it, because it is the addicts who generally come to the attention of treatment and criminal justice personnel.

HEROIN USE AND DEPENDENCE

Population-based surveys covering the use of all illicit drugs often do not assess dependence or addiction at all. Estimates based on such surveys indicate that only about 1 percent of the U.S. population has ever tried heroin. The few studies that have measured dependence find that less than half of this 1 percent who try heroin ever develop dependence. The percentage currently dependent is not known precisely. Nor is it known what proportion of those currently dependent would qualify for methadone maintenance programs by having been daily users for a year or longer and unable to cease on their own or with medical supervision. But the proportion of the population who could be candidates for methadone maintenance must be smaller than the 0.5 percent who have ever been dependent. We discuss below some findings from epidemiologic studies that put upper bounds on the number of addicts in the population.

Available epidemiological data on heroin use and dependence, coupled with data from other sources about the addict population, provide a background for placing methadone treatment in context and answering a number of specific questions that affect the committee's charge.

Prevalence of Heroin Use

While the use of other drugs has varied considerably over time, the number of persons who reported that they had ever used heroin, a number which soared about 1969, appears to have been quite stable since then at just below 1 percent of the general population. This stability is demonstrated in Lloyd Johnston's graphs, showing results from Monitoring the Future, a nationwide longitudinal, cohort study (Johnston, et al., 1993). In this study, each year 12,000 to 18,000 adolescents, selected from senior classes in a national sample of high schools, are surveyed; of those graduating from 1978 to 1991, representative samples of 2,400 have been selected for follow-up each year. The 2,400 are randomly divided in half and 1,200 are followed every two years on even years, 1,200 every two years on odd years. Thus, the sample of young adults being surveyed in recent years includes every age from 19 to 32.

This study found a stable rate of heroin use by young adults initially surveyed as high school seniors since 1986 (see Figure 3-1). The low flat curve for heroin use contrasts with that for crack cocaine use, which has been declining since 1986. In this study, Johnston and colleagues found rates of ever having tried heroin differed with age—1.2 percent of the 18-year-olds compared to 3 percent of those 31–32 years old. Interestingly, none of the older group with heroin experience admitted any heroin use in the year before the interview. In no age group did the proportion using in the last month rise above 0.3 percent, and it was less than 0.1 percent in those 25 or older. The fact that less than a quarter of those who report ever having used heroin also report use in the last month suggests either that use by high school seniors does not often lead to dependence or that dependence is typically brief, or both. Since the proportion of subjects who used any heroin at all in the last month is less than 0.2 percent, the proportion currently addicted to heroin has to be below that figure. However, this conclusion should be interpreted with caution, as persons who reach the senior year of high school, having shown a capacity to manage their school careers, may be less susceptible to the serious consequences of heroin use than others their age not in school.

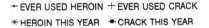

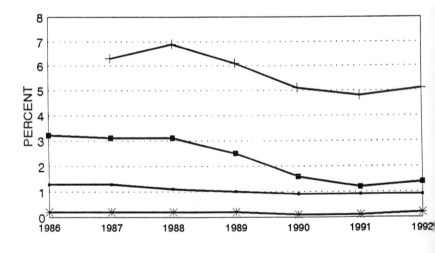

FIGURE 3-1 Changes in drug use over time by young adults—heroin compared to crack cocaine. SOURCE: Johnston et al. (1993).

Another important epidemiological study of drug use is the National Household Survey, which interviews persons 12 years old and older in a national sample of household residents every year or two. In the 1992 National

Household Survey, the proportion of interviewed household members who had ever used heroin was 0.9 percent and use in the last year was 0.2 percent. The age group with the highest lifetime rate of having ever used heroin was the 26–34-year-olds (1.6 percent) and of having recent use was the 18–25 year-olds (0.5 percent). These data support Johnston's finding that most of those who ever used heroin no longer use it.

From Use to Dependence

Neither Monitoring the Future nor the National Household Survey assesses dependence on or addiction to heroin, only the amount of use. Indeed, population surveys that provide rates of dependence on heroin are scarce. Even in these surveys, when the population sampled is limited to household residents, questions can be raised about the prevalence estimates for dependence because not all addicts live in households and those in households may be unwilling to be interviewed. Therefore, estimates of the number of heroin-dependent individuals based on household surveys must be considered minimum estimates.

Four general population studies have assessed dependence on heroin as well as use. In a small study (N = 235) of young African-American men born and brought up in St. Louis (conducted in 1965), 13 percent had used heroin, with use generally beginning between ages 16 and 23 (around 1950). Ten percent of the sample, or 79 percent of the men who reported using heroin, said they had become addicted to it (Robins and Murphy, 1967), by which they meant they were heavy users and had experienced withdrawal symptoms. In 1973, in a follow-up of a random sample of Army enlisted men (N = 900) who had been in Vietnam at the height of the heroin epidemic there in 1970–1971, about 44 percent reported having tried an opiate while there, and 20 percent became addicted, again defined as heavy use plus persistent withdrawal symptoms when they stopped. Thus they had a 45 percent risk of dependence if they used (Robins, 1974). In 1982, the Epidemiological Catchment Area (ECA), a large study of mental disorders in the general population, interviewed 18,000 persons 18 years of age and older, including the institutionalized. When weighted to make the sample representative of the total U.S. population over 18, 1.3 percent had tried heroin six times or more and 48 percent of these more-than-experimental users had become dependent according to DSM-III criteria (Anthony and Helzer, 1991). Finally, in the recent National Comorbidity Study, 8,098 household residents aged 15–54 were asked if they had ever used heroin even once; one percent had used, and only 23 percent of users qualified as ever dependent according to DSM-III-R criteria (NCS, 1994). The last two studies, which are studies of the general adult population, find lifetime rates of heroin dependence of 0.6 percent and 0.2 percent. The proportion who are candidates for methadone treatment, because their dependence was severe enough to qualify as addiction and for whom the addiction is currently active, must be smaller than these figures.

The first of these four studies was conducted in 1965, the most recent in 1992. Although they differ in populations studied, methods of sampling, and questions asked, they agree that many who try heroin do not become dependent on it. The rates of use and dependence suggest that the risk of becoming dependent if heroin is tried may have declined over the 30 years the studies span.

However, there is no guarantee that the stability (or possible decline) of dependence among heroin users will continue. In the late 1980s, the price of heroin fell sharply and the purity of street heroin rose. Although most heroin addicts use injection into the vein as their method of ingestion, the quality of heroin in some areas of the country is now high enough to allow smoking or snorting as a route of administration, thus removing a major barrier to heroin use. These changes may lead to both an increase in users and a higher probability that users will become addicted.

How Persistent Is Heroin Dependence?

Although estimates of the typical duration of dependence are not precise, these studies suggest that dependence often ends without treatment. The study of young African-American St. Louis men found only 3 out of 22 self-described one-time "addicts" still using heroin in their early thirties, although only 4 had any treatment. Only 12 percent of the Vietnam veterans who reported having been "addicted" in Vietnam reported relapse in the first three years after their return to the United States, and these self-reports were confirmed by almost uniformly negative urine tests for opiates at 1 and 3 years after their return. In the ECA, which evaluated dependence according to DSM-III criteria, the St. Louis sample was asked whether problems had been experienced with each drug used in the last year. Among the St. Louis ECA subjects who had ever been dependent on heroin, only 5 percent reported having had any of the symptoms of heroin dependence in the current year.

The above paragraph in no way denies the importance, and the needs, of the significant group of those who become dependent and progress to addiction and who find it impossible to quit without help. This addict population is a subset of the general heroin user population and differs from it in important ways.

Information about the addict group is available from several long-term natural history studies of addicts known to treatment or the courts, including

Vaillant (1973), Simpson et al. (1986), and Hser et al. (1993). This last study followed 581 male heroin addicts from about 1962–1964, when the average age of this group was 25.4 years and they had been addicted nearly six years, through 1986, when they had an average age of 47.6 years. Over this 24-year period, 28 percent had died. At interview in 1986, 18 percent were incarcerated, 23 percent had urines positive for heroin, only 29 percent were urine negative, and only 20 percent reported having been heroin-abstinent during the previous three years.

The Hser findings were similar to those of the other two studies, which found that death, incarceration, or continued addiction was the course of the majority of addicts identified in treatment or criminal justice settings. Once heroin addiction is established, in many cases even for a relatively short period, it tends to persist and most addicts relapse repeatedly. It is this group of chronic addicts for whom methadone programs provide opportunities for living a productive life.

Age, Gender, and Ethnicity

General population surveys identify some relationships between individual demographic characteristics and heroin dependence. Most of these relationships are confirmed in special population studies (see below), but some change when only the treated addict population is considered.

Age

Heroin-dependent individuals in the 1990s are mostly under 40 years of age. Their youth can be explained in three ways: First, few people now over 50 have ever tried heroin, which became generally available around 1970 but has been initiated almost exclusively before age 30, thus leaving out persons over 30 when it first appeared. Second, the death rate among heroin addicts is high, decimating those who continue their addiction for 10 years or longer. Third, chances of recovery increase with age, so that those who try to quit are increasingly successful as they mature. Thus, heroin dependence typically began in the early 20s among persons born after 1945 and eventuated either in death or recovery by age 40.

Gender

Gender is less strongly related to use and dependence than is age, but the relationship is still substantial. There is good agreement across studies that heroin dependence is predominantly male. Rates in men were 2.5 times that in women in the National Comorbidity Study. In the ECA, male rates were almost 5 times that in women. However, the ECA found that dependent women are slightly more likely to recover than men (55 percent versus 47 percent).

Ethnicity

Heroin is somewhat more popular with African-Americans than whites, although differences are small. In the National Household Survey, 1 percent of African-Americans and 0.9 percent of whites had tried heroin. Among high school seniors followed into adulthood, 2 percent of African-Americans and 1.2 percent of whites 26–32 years old had ever tried heroin (Johnston et al., 1993). The association of minority status is much less pronounced than the association of either age or gender with the use of heroin. There were too few minority users in the ECA to allow reliable comparisons of races with respect to the chance that users would become dependent.

What Other Substances Do Heroin Users Consume?

Every population study in the last 30 years has found that heroin-dependent persons typically use and become dependent on a variety of other substances, both legal and illegal, in addition to heroin. In the Vietnam study for example, those who used heroin after their return to the United States on average used 8 different illicit drugs. Men dependent on heroin were asked what their *main* drug was after their return from Vietnam; 40 percent named alcohol, marijuana, or some drug *other* than heroin. Among heroin-dependent persons in the ECA, conducted in the early 1980s, more than 40 percent also had problems with cannabis and sedatives and almost as many had problems with stimulants (39 percent). The ECA showed that 48 percent of heroin-dependent persons were also alcohol-dependent.

The main national shift in consumption of illicit drugs in the 1980s is certainly to cocaine. The 1982 ECA sample contained 6.5 times as many heroin users as users of cocaine. In 1992, the National Comorbidity Study found the relationship had reversed—there were over 6 times as many cocaine users as heroin users.

These results suggest that heroin-addicted persons in treatment will have dependencies on a variety of other substances and that problems with drugs other than heroin may be as responsible as heroin for their distress and maladjustment. Data from community, arrestee, and treatment populations presented below confirm these results. Indeed, the presence of severe problems due to drug use is an increasingly frequent characteristic of heroin addicts, according to clinicians.

Other Medical and Social Problems of Heroin-Dependent Persons

Heroin-dependent persons typically have a variety of psychiatric, medical, and social problems in addition to their substance dependence. As compared to persons their own age and sex, heroin-dependent individuals in the ECA had an excess of depression and other serious psychiatric disorders. ECA data for the 248 men under 40 who ever met the criteria for heroin dependence showed dramatic rates of comorbidities compared with the remaining 3,800 men in the same age group. Depression was found in 19 percent of the former compared with 4 percent of the remainder; schizophrenic symptoms in 9 percent versus 2 percent; panic disorder in 5 percent versus 2 percent; and a manic episode in 4 percent versus 1 percent of other young men. Whether or not these disorders are the result of the heroin dependence, or independent of it, it is clear that persons dependent on heroin need psychiatric assessment and treatment.

The heroin-dependent person frequently has many medical problems in addition to his or her dependence. Some of these problems stem from the way in which heroin is administered and its illegal status, rather than from the effects of heroin itself. It is injection that accounts primarily for infections, hepatitis, and AIDS. It is the illegal status of heroin that accounts for the elevated risks of homicide and injury associated with its purchase and sale, and for overdose death or poisoning due to variations in the strength and purity of the drug as purchased on the street. Methadone maintenance treatment makes a major contribution to the addict's health and to public health in general by eliminating or reducing injection and the purchase and sale of heroin in the illicit market, and by substituting a drug of known strength and quality for street drugs.

Despite their liability to ill health as a result of infections or the drug itself, heroin-dependent persons are not heavy users of routine or primary medical services. In the ECA, heroin-dependent persons were no more likely than others to have seen a doctor in the last 6 months. When these individuals do seek medical care, it is often at hospital emergency rooms and when their medical problems have reached an advanced stage. Thus, dependent persons, and certainly heroin addicts among them, appear to be a particularly medically underserved population.

Heroin-dependent persons have a number of social problems, including difficulty in holding jobs, obeying laws, maintaining stable marriages, making and keeping friends, and functioning as caring and responsible parents. These difficulties are related to the fact that getting and using drugs leaves little time for other activities. In addition, heroin addicts commit a large number of crimes in order to support their addiction.

Many who become heroin-dependent had, while still children and before any drug use, behaviors that forecast adult social problems in non-drug-users as well as in heroin addicts. For example, there was frequently a childhood and early adolescent history of school problems and truancy, delinquency, drinking, lying, running away from home, and fighting. The fact that these early behaviors predict adult social problems independent of drug dependence means that once the heroin addiction is controlled through methadone treatment, the addict's social problems are likely to decline but not vanish. Many addicts will still be socially incompetent and continue to be involved in illegal behaviors, because they had these tendencies before their addiction.

When considering what methadone treatment is likely to accomplish, then, it is important to remember that the heroin-dependent person who has progressed to addiction brings many medical and social problems to the treatment setting, in addition to addiction, that pose a challenge to the treatment system going well beyond treating drug addiction. Many clinicians believe that these other problems have become more severe in today's patient.

How Likely Are Heroin Addicts to Use Treatment?

What proportion of all addicts enter treatment? According to self-report data in the ECA, 37 percent of heroin-dependent persons have ever attended a drug treatment program, a proportion that does not vary with age. Dependent men, on the other hand, were less likely to attend than dependent women (32 percent versus 51 percent). But the greatest difference was found by ethnic background. Only 28 percent of white heroin-dependent persons had attended a specialized drug treatment program, although 50 percent of minority heroin-dependent persons had done so (calculated for the committee from ECA tapes). The result is that minorities are more overrepresented in treated populations than in the total user population.

What characteristics of an addict are associated with the decision to enter treatment? Those persons who enter treatment are older and have been more severely addicted for a longer time than heroin-dependent persons who do not enter treatment. Although treated addicts, like the general population of heroin users, are disproportionately young males, this disproportion is less striking than in the general heroin population. The greater representation of older addicts in treatment is explained both by the fact that it is only after some years that the disadvantages of addiction relative to its pleasures become apparent and drive the addict to seek help, and by the fact that the first treatment episode often fails, which means that the treated population includes a large number of repeaters, i.e., those who have relapsed to heroin use and have then returned to treatment. The greater representation of female addicts in treatment may be explained by the fact that, in general, women are more likely than men to seek medical care (Fiorentine and Anglin, 1993).

CHARACTERISTICS OF UNTREATED AND TREATED HEROIN ADDICTS

This section shifts the focus from population-based surveys to surveys of heroin addicts. Empirical data are presented that characterize what is known about contemporary populations of untreated and treated addicts.

If one moves from examining the characteristics of users and addicts that are demarcated by general population epidemiological studies, which have been discussed earlier, to characteristics as demarcated by epidemiological studies specific to addicts, then the chronicity of addiction and the dysfunctional nature of addict lifestyles becomes quite clear. Table 3-1 provides such addict-specific information by drawing on data from samples or subsamples within two multiple-site national studies. The first is the National AIDS Demonstration Research (NADR) program, funded by NIDA in 59 sites across the nation. Results from a NADR subsample were among the most salient in indicating the large proportion of heroin addicts who have never received formal treatment. The second is the Drug Use Forecasting (DUF) program, funded by NIJ for calendar year 1990 in 24 cities across the United States. Each quarter, DUF staff selects booked arrestees and interviews them about their drug use histories. Unlike most other surveys of addicts, DUF also requests voluntary urine samples—which are provided in 85–90 percent of cases—which are objectively tested for the presence of 10 drugs. Given their extensive geographic coverage, access to heroin addicts, and large sample sizes, these two studies (which are also discussed in Chapter 4) provide very useful data related to untreated and treated heroin addicts.

The interpretation of the data provided in Table 3-1 should focus primarily on the pattern of responses within each study, and only limited comparisons should be made across the studies. This is necessary because study methodologies access different samples, and define somewhat different measures for the variables represented.

The first study, the NADR study, included a fairly large subsample of primary heroin addicts (about 16,500) accessed through nontraditional access mechanisms (i.e., they were not drawn from treatment programs or criminal justice populations). The three groups within this subsample are large, each exceeding 5,000, being evenly distributed across addicts who report no treatment history (34 percent), those who report a treatment history exclusive of methadone (32 percent), and those who report any methadone maintenance history (34 percent). Data from this study recapitulate a number of the findings reported earlier for general population studies of heroin users and addicts. These include the finding that the proportion of women among those reporting methadone maintenance histories is higher than the proportion of women among those reporting any nonmethadone treatment history or no treatment history. While proportions of African-Americans are equivalent across all three groups at about 42–44 percent, the proportion of Hispanics decreases steadily across the three groups and the proportion of whites increases steadily. The mean age also increases across the three groups from 33 years in the group reporting no treatment history to 37 years in those reporting some prior exposure to methadone maintenance. Similarly, the proportions of those over 30 years old in each group increase steadily to a maximum of 87 percent in the methadone maintenance treatment group. In contrast to the no-treatment-history group, those with a treatment history, particularly those with a methadone maintenance history, report more prior contact with the criminal justice system and have longer reported years of addiction. The methadone group reports higher rates of prior treatment than the nonmethdone treatment group. The methadone maintenance group reports slightly less employment before interview, and slightly more criminal involvement, than the other groups. Rates of cocaine use are similar across all three groups, while rates of marijuana use are less in the methadone maintenance group.

The DUF data cover approximately the same period as do the NADR data. The sample size reported for 1990 is reasonably large, at about 3,000 cases. As might be expected with an arrestee population, over 60 percent report no treatment history. A caution in interpreting the DUF data is important here. Any arrestee who reported prior opiate dependence or whose urine was opiate positive at the time of interview was included in the opiate user or addict category. Therefore, that group may include some few opiate users who were not addicted. Furthermore, this data base did not distinguish between methadone maintenance and other types of drug treatment.

Replicating earlier patterns described in this chapter, the sample shows that those reporting a treatment history are somewhat more likely to be women, to be white, and to be older. Rates of reported legal income in the period before interview are surprisingly high and involvement in criminal activity is significant, with the treated group somewhat less employed and more criminally involved. Use of other substances is similar across the two groups, but the treated group reports slightly more cocaine use, and slightly less marijuana use.

In sum, opiate users accessing treatment have more extensive histories of opiate addiction, have more prior treatment failures, and are marginal in terms of employment, criminal activities, and polysubstance abuse. The population of untreated and previously treated opiate addicts together comprises the pool of active users who may need, may seek, and may utilize methadone maintenance treatment. This brings us to our third source of information about heroin use, dependence, addiction, and treatment: addicts now in methadone maintenance treatment.

METHADONE PATIENT CHARACTERISTICS

The following section presents data on historical tends and current characteristics of those heroin addicts now in methadone maintenance treatment. We examine most closely methadone maintenance clients, and briefly describe methadone detoxification clients. As noted above, there are some significant differences between the general heroin-addicted population and the patient population. Overall, addicts who enter into a methadone treatment program either maintenance or detoxification, are more desperate, more physically and mentally ill, poorer, and more disabled than the general addict population. In addition there are regional differences in patient characteristics as well as differences between patients in publicly funded treatment programs, and in programs relying on private (usually client paid fee-for-service) funds.

Historical Trends

Three nationwide studies of drug abusers entering treatment have been conducted that provide information as to historical trends in methadone maintenance treatment admissions over the last three decades. The first of these was a series of studies collectively called the Drug Abuse Reporting Program (DARP) research on drug treatment admissions during the years 1969 through 1973. The second series of studies was known as the Treatment Outcomes Prospective Studies (TOPS), which yielded characteristics of patients entering methadone maintenance during the years 1979 through 1981 (see Flynn et al., 1994). The most recent nationwide study, known as the Drug Abuse Treatment Outcome Studies (DATOS), examined methadone patient characteristics for the years 1991 through 1993 (see Flynn et al., 1994). Finally, special computer runs in 1993 by SAMHSA's Office of Applied Studies detail characteristics of methadone maintenance admissions for the 26 states reporting admissions for calendar year 1992. Table 3-2 shows basic characteristics of methadone maintenance patient across the time periods represented by the data.

TABLE 3-1 Characteristics of Heroin Users and Addicts at Percentage Occurrences Within Untreated and Treated Groups

Characteristic	NADR Sample (total N = ~16,500)			DUF Sample (total N = ~3,000)	
	No Treatment (N = 5,542; 34% of total)	Some Nonmethadone Treatment History (N = 5,296; 32% of total)	Some Methadone Maintenance History (N = 5,662; 34% of total)	No Treatment History (N = 1,092; 63% of total)	Any Treatment History (N = 1,095; 37% of total)
Female	27	25	32	32	38
African-American	43	42	44	48	41
Hispanic	42	36	30	25	22
Mean age[a]	33	34	37	31	34
Over 30-years old	66	72	87	57	70
High school graduate	48	56	61	58	61
Ever married	—	—	—	—	48
Prior incarceration	75	85	91	—	—
Years addicted[a]	12	14	18	—	—

3 or more prior	0	43	77	—	—
Court referred	—	—	—	—	—
On legal supervision	23	28	30	—	—
Employed	28	28	28	71^b	65^b
Criminal activity	44	49	53	30^c	42^c
Cocaine use[d]	81	84	79	70	76
Marijuana use[d]	39	37	28	28	22

NOTE: NADR = National AIDS Demonstration Research programs; interviewers were heroin addicts not accessed through treatment programs or the criminal justice system. DUF = Drug Use Forecasting program; interviewers were arrestees categorized as opiate users or addicts. NADR data are for 1989–1990; DUF data are for 1990.

[a]Data in this row are mean years.
[b]Percentage reporting legal income sources in past month.
[c]Percentage reporting illegal income sources in past month.
[d]Reported as a secondary drug problem.

SOURCE: Complied from data from the NADR program and the DUF program by Mel Widawski, Senior Statistician at the Drug Abuse Research Center of the University of California, Los Angeles.

In examining the data presented in Table 3-2 it should be kept in mind that the first study depicted, DARP for the years 1969–1973, occurred primarily in the years before federal regulations were instituted (see chapter 5). The second and third studies, TOPS and DATOS, occurred after the institution of federal, and subsequently State, regulations, at approximately 10-year intervals. The final column includes data from the Client Data System (CDS) maintained currently by the Substance Abuse Mental Health Services Administration, Office of Applied Studies. These data are not from a research study, as were the prior three, but are instead from a drug treatment admission monitoring system, which is discussed in more detail below. Of most importance for methadone regulation purposes are the DARP, TOPS, and DATOS study. The CDS information is presented primarily as a confirmation of the accuracy with which the DATOS sample represents the full population of methadone admissions for about the same period.

The following changes across the three studies are worth noting. First, the proportion of women in methadone treatment increased steadily from 22 percent in the DARP studies to 39 percent in the DATOS studies. Second, the proportion of African-Americans decreased from 58 percent in DARP to 28 percent in DATOS; the proportion of Hispanics grew from 10 percent in DARP to 24 percent in DATOS; and the percent of those who are white has increased by approximately nine years across the three studies, and the proportion of patients over 30 years old reached 80 percent in the DATOS studies. In the DARP studies the average years addicted for methadone admissions was 9–10; this rose to 13 by the early 1990s (i.e., by the time of the DATOS studies). The proportion receiving previous treatment was approximately 50 percent during the DARP period, a rate which rose to about 75 percent for the subsequent study periods. Similarly the proportion with three or more treatments was only 13 percent for DARP, increasing to 44 percent and 40 percent for the subsequent two studies respectively. The percentage of admissions with prior incarceration histories remained in excess of 50 percent, and the percentage under legal supervision at program entry varied but represented a significant minority over all three study periods, as did the level of criminal involvement among patients. The percentage of employed patients dropped somewhat from the DARP period to the subsequent two study periods, demonstrating the marginal employability of more recent methadone admission populations. Cocaine use was 25–35 percent of the admission population in the DARP and TOPS studies and nearly 50 percent of the DATOS admissions. Marijuana use as a secondary drug problem declined in recent study periods, as did use of alcohol.

The similarity in the patient characteristics across the three series of studies is quite striking. Generally, patients entering methadone maintenance treatment are dysfunctional in a number of behavioral domains, show long histories of chronic addiction, have serious involvement with the criminal justice system, and typically access treatment repeatedly after their first episode is complete.

Current Patient Characteristics

As of December 1993, there were 759 methadone maintenance programs in the United States (FDA tabulation). These programs typically maintain a census of some 115,000 patients. Only one national data base, the Client Data System mentioned above, which is maintained by SAMHSA's Office of Applied Studies, contains information of definitive patient characteristics, and the data collected are limited. Even so, the CDS provides a great deal of information about the annual number of admissions. However, its data are more complete for publicly funded treatment programs than for private, proprietary programs; comprehensive information about all treatment programs is not available at this time. Similar limitations characterize the California Alcohol and Drug Data System, whose data are used in further discussions below.

The CDS is based upon admissions data on methadone patients in treatment programs as reported by 31 of the 42 reporting states.[1] (During 1992, as discussed earlier and shown on Table 3-2, 26 states reported admission for methadone maintenance treatment. Reports and numbers of admissions for detoxification treatment are counted separately. See further discussion below.) This data base offers some information about the age, sex, and race of patients upon entry into a treatment program, and allows discovering regional differences. However, in any one year a single patient may have more than one admission reported to CDS. To reduce the error introduced by counting patients multiple times, admissions designated as transfers are excluded from consideration. Still, patients may drop out of a program and later return for a new episode of treatment in the same or a different program. Data are presented below in three areas: first, any admission to methadone treatment; second, methadone detoxification; and, finally, methadone maintenance.

---

[1] Appreciation is expressed to the SAMHSA Office of Applied Studies for providing special runs on primary heroin users assigned to methadone treatment.

TABLE 3-2 Methadone Maintenance Patient Characteristics as Percentage Occurrences Within Programs, 1969–1993

Characteristic	DARP, 1969–1973 (N = 11,023; 34 programs)	TOPS, 1969–1973 (N = 4,184; 17 programs)	DATOS, 1969–73 (N = 1,540; 29 programs)	CDS (1992) (N = 41,509; 26 states reporting)
Female	22	32	39	36
African-American	58	37	28	33
Hispanic	25	21	24	27
White	15	20	25	25
Mean age[a]	28	31	37	—
Over 30-years old	30	40	80	79
High school graduate	37	48	64	69
Ever married	46	56	69	51
Prior incarceration	50	80	63	—
Years addicted[a]	9–10	12	13	—
3 or more prior treatments	13	44	40	36
Court referred	7	3	2	6
On legal supervision (pre-interview)	30	18	21	—

[Employed]	30	24	16	21
Criminal activity	47–52	33	48	—
Cocaine use[b]	<34	28	42	52
Marijuana use[b]	<55	55	18	Court referred

NOTE: DARP = Drug Abuse Reporting Program; TOPS = Treatment Outcomes Prospective Studies; DATOS = Drug Abuse Treatment Outcome Studies; CDS = Client Data System maintained by SAMHSA's office of Applied Studies (OAS).

[a]Data in this row are mean years.
[b]Reported as secondary drug problem.

SOURCE: Sampson et al. (1976) (DARP); Hubbard et al. (1989) and Flynn et al. (1994) (TOPS and DATOS); special computer runs by SAMHSA-OAS (CDS).

Methadone in Drug Treatment: General

Overall, in fiscal year 1992, 97,519 admissions for both detoxification and methadone maintenance were reported by 31 of the 42 reporting states as having been assigned to receive methadone as part of treatment.[2] Although methadone maintenance is the treatment for persistent opiate dependence with the best evidence of effectiveness, it appears to be infrequently utilized in many states treatment systems. Even in those states where such programs exist, the utilization of methadone treatment by opiate-dependent individuals varies dramatically. Five of the reporting jurisdictions (California, District of Columbia, New Jersey, New York, and Rhode Island) predominate in the methadone maintenance treatment data, each accounting for more than 10 percent of the nation's methadone treatment admissions. Eight states reported fewer than 100 admissions. Nationally, admissions to methadone maintenance or detoxification were 64 percent male, and 46 percent were white, 12 percent African-American, and 38 percent Hispanic. The modal ages were 35 to 44 years of age (44 percent of admissions). Among the 23 states reporting at least 100 admissions, 47 percent of those admitted had three or more prior treatment episodes, and 42 percent reported that cocaine was a secondary substance of abuse.

Of particular interest are the differences between states in the treatment settings that use methadone. For example, in the state of Pennsylvania, 26 percent of admissions for treatment utilizing methadone occurred in hospital inpatient detoxification settings, a considerably greater percentage than in New York and Texas, where only 10 percent and 14 percent, respectively, of admissions were for inpatient detoxification. Most other states appeared not to use methadone in inpatient or residential settings at all. Minnesota is an exception; there, methadone was used extensively in residential settings (68 percent of admissions—19 percent hospital-based, 49 percent nonhospital). Generally, methadone is provided in ambulatory outpatient settings, but states differ significantly here as well. All of Connecticut's methadone admissions were into intensive outpatient programs, as were 32 percent of admissions in Minnesota and 10 percent in North Carolina. Most other states, however, reported that nonintensive outpatient services only were utilized, or that outpatient detoxification services were utilized. In this last regard, state policies again differed. For example, in California, 81 percent of all methadone admissions were to outpatient detoxification programs and only 17 percent

---

[2] This annual estimate of admissions is a count of new *and* repeat entries to treatment. Thus, it is not a measure of incidence of admissions new to treatment. I differs from the 115,000 census figure of treated patients, which is a point prevalence count of all patients typically in methadone maintenance treatment any one time.

were to methadone maintenance programs. This pattern was also true in Hawaii (78 percent and 17 percent). By contrast, 97 percent of admissions in Illinois were to methadone maintenance programs, as were 88 percent in the District of Columbia, and 82 percent in New York. These figures highlight the variation in the use methadone treatment across states (see also chapter 6).

Use of Methadone in Detoxification

Of the 42,615 admissions to detoxification treatment reported by 12 states in fiscal year 1992, the great majority (86 percent) were in California. New Jersey accounted for 10 percent and Maryland for 2 percent. No other state reporting to the CDS had more than 300 admissions for detoxification. Of the nationwide admissions for detoxification treatment, 65 percent were male; 43 percent were white, 18 percent African-American, and 35 percent Hispanic. The high percentage of Hispanic admissions probably reflects the domination of the detoxification figures by the California data. Forty-three percent were between 35 and 44 years of age.

Use of Methadone in Maintenance Treatment

The 41,509 admissions reported by 26 states for methadone maintenance also showed a different distribution by state. In fiscal year 1992, New York led with 33 percent of the total, followed by California with 19 percent, New Jersey with 8 percent, Massachusetts with 7 percent, and the District of Columbia with 6 percent. No other state reported more than 2,500 admissions, with a range of 7 to 2,409.

The gender distribution was similar to that seen in detoxification admissions, with males accounting for 64 percent. The ethnic breakdown was somewhat different: 38 percent white, 33 percent African-American, and 27 percent Hispanic. As with detoxification admissions, 46 percent were between 35 and 44 years of age.

Contrast Between Detoxification and Maintenance Patient Admissions

Characteristics of detoxification and maintenance patient admissions are similar, except in the following areas: There are more repeaters among those detoxified, where 42 percent reported 5 or more prior treatment episodes compared to 19 percent for methadone maintenance admissions.

Referrals by the criminal justice system account for a smaller proportion of detoxification admissions (1 percent) than of maintenance (6 percent). In fact, referrals to detoxification are almost entirely self-referrals (93 percent). More of those admitted for detoxification than for maintenance reported injection as the primary route of administration (91 percent versus 74 percent). Inhalation is reported by only 8 percent of those admitted for detoxification admissions compared with 24 percent of those admitted for maintenance (probably because New York and New Jersey provide maintenance treatment to large numbers of addicts and it is in these two states where inhalation, or snorting, is on the rise).

Nearly all persons admitted for detoxification (98 percent) are daily users of opiates compared to 85 percent of maintenance admissions. Forty percent of those admitted for detoxification report secondary substance abuse, and 30 percent report cocaine use. Among those admitted for maintenance, the corresponding figures are 57 percent and 52 percent. Persons admitted for maintenance treatment report more psychiatric problems (7 percent) than those admitted for detoxification (1 percent). More women admitted to maintenance treatment are pregnant (10 percent) than are women admitted to detoxification (1 percent).

Only about one-third of methadone patients are currently employed, whether admitted to detoxification or maintenance treatment. Finally, while more of those admitted for maintenance than for detoxification admissions have been married (61 percent versus 39 percent), only one in five in either group is currently married.

To provide more detailed information on the use of methadone in maintenance treatment, we present data from two states with large maintenance populations, New York and California.

Maintenance Patients in New York State; 1992

Some one-third of the methadone maintenance treatment population of the United States is in New York State programs. The census of patients in these programs as of January 1, 1992, was 39,340; two-thirds were male.

Unlike the general addict population, two-thirds of these methadone patients were over age 35. As of January 1994, the mean age of the treated population was 39.5 years—39.6 for males and 36.9 for females.

Heroin use generally began during their teens. Fifty-seven percent reported beginning heroin use by age nineteen; 20 percent started use by age fifteen. Conversely, less than 10 percent reported starting heroin use after age twenty nine.

With regard to race-ethnic status, these New York State male methadone patients were almost evenly composed of three groups: African-American (27 percent); Hispanic (36 percent); and white (35 percent). The distribution among female patients was still more evenly balanced: African-American (34 percent); Hispanic (34 percent); and white (31 percent).

Almost all (96 percent) of the patients in methadone maintenance programs in New York State reported that heroin was their primary drug of abuse before treatment. Interestingly, unlike any other state, almost a thousand patients reported that street methadone was their chief drug of abuse prior to treatment; use of street methadone, then, accounted for some 3 percent of admissions.

Data concerning route of drug administration for the 1992 New York State active treatment population (approximately 30,000) indicate that intravenous use (injecting) has declined from prior years. (NIDA has established the following routes of administration for minimum data set purposes: oral, smoking, inhalation (snorting), injection, and other.) Of the male methadone maintenance patients, 74 percent reported at admission that injecting was their common route of use, 24 percent reported inhalation (snorting), and 2 percent reported other routes (oral, smoking, other). The females, however, were less likely than the males to be intravenous drug users: among female patients, 66 percent reported injecting, 24 percent inhalation, and 15 percent other routes. In both sexes, primarily intravenous use has notably declined in the past several years, from 82 percent of admissions in 1986 to 57 percent in 1992 (approximately 11,000).

In addition to a long history of opiate abuse, most of these methadone maintenance patients have abused other drugs as well. Overall, the secondary drugs of abuse for males and females were quite similar; over half of both male and female patients report cocaine use.

Most (75 percent) of the methadone maintenance patients in treatment in New York State had one or more prior treatments for drug abuse. These prior treatments included detoxification and therapeutic communities, as well as methadone maintenance and other modalities.

Maintenance Patients in California, 1992

The California Alcohol and Drug Data System (CADDS) contains data from all methadone treatment programs except those in Department of Veterans Affairs hospitals. The system includes the data required for reporting to CDS (see discussion above) as well as other information collected for state use. California limits the number of methadone detoxification slots, and limits Medi-Cal reimbursement to a maximum of 21 days per detoxification treatment episode. Admissions for methadone detoxification during calendar year 1992 were 30,981 for men and 15,924 for women. Discharges were 30,806 and 15,826, respectively, resulting in a January 1, 1993, census of 1,209 men and

666 women. (These treatment census figures are substantially below the licensed detoxification capacity due to lags in reporting by some large counties.)

In California, detoxification patients are similar to maintenance patients, except they are more often male. Women admitted to detoxification report pregnancy less often than those admitted for maintenance. Detoxification admissions report fewer prior treatment episodes than do maintenance admissions. The differences are due, in part, to state regulations that require at least two prior treatment failures for maintenance admissions, but not for detoxification admissions. In addition, high rates of prior treatment among those admitted for detoxification are partly explained by the way treatment is reimbursed in California. Although limited in length, detoxification is fully reimbursed (i.e., no copayment) by Medi-Cal for the majority of admissions, while maintenance treatment is reimbursed only in specific cases, such as pregnant women, HIV-positive patients, and limited other groups.

As of January 1, 1992, there were 15,896 patients being served by California methadone maintenance programs. This group was 57 percent male, for whom the average age was 38.7 years with three-fourths being age 33 or older. For females, the average age was 34.9 years with three-fourths being age 30 or older. Whites made up the largest proportion of clients for both males (53 percent) and females (61 percent), while Hispanics made up the next largest proportion (35 percent for males and 26 percent for females). African-Americans constituted the vast majority of the remaining admissions.

The majority of clients were "self-referred" into treatment: 83 percent of males and 78 percent of females. Referrals from alcohol/drug programs or from the court/criminal justice system accounted for just under 10 percent each for both males and females. Approximately 20 percent of both males and females had some type of involvement with the criminal justice program at the time of admission. One-third of the males and 41 percent of females had less than 12 years of education. Employment (including part time) was 13.6 percent among males and 7.1 percent among females.

Finally, as is to be expected because current state regulations require at least two treatment failures before maintenance admission, except for emergency admissions, which require no prior treatment failures, only 1 percent of the males and 1.8 percent of the females reported no prior treatment. This is in contrast to New York methadone maintenance patients, 25 percent of whom have reported no prior treatment.

Nearly all methadone maintenance clients claimed heroin as their primary drug (98 percent for both males and females), and injection as the main route of administration (about 96 percent) for both. A large proportion were daily users (85.9 percent and 82.9 percent for males and females, respectively). A very small proportion of the sample reported street methadone as their main drug (0.2 percent for both males and females). The average age of first opiate use was 20.9 for males and 21.5 for females, with half of the males beginning use on or before age 19 and half of the females beginning use on or before age 20.

Just over half of the males and about three-fifths of the females were using cocaine as a secondary drug, with over half using it on a daily basis. Of those using cocaine, 12.2 percent of the males and 18.6 percent of the females were using crack. Alcohol was the next most popular secondary drug of abuse among males (24.4 percent) and females (16.8 percent).

Differences Between New York and California

The previous paragraphs described in detail the methadone maintenance data for the two states that together serve the majority of methadone maintenance patients in the United States. The data from New York and California allow some summary data to be extracted which highlight the differences between the two systems. Although the specific data are informative, a contrast of some overall system parameters indicates the extent to which state and local government policy affects treatment availability, utilization, and outcome.

Table 3-3 shows the most recent data available for both states with respect to their methadone maintenance patient census as of January 1 in 1992 and 1993; their rates of admission and discharge during the year; the percentage of system growth over the year; and the rate of patient movement into and out of treatment, measure as a "turnover rate" (calculated by dividing the total 1992 discharges by the January 1, 1992, patient census).

Before discussing specific differences, a comparison of each state's overall government policies toward methadone is informative. New York State, particularly New York City, has been troubled by heroin addiction since World War II, and has the longest history of comprehensive government-sponsored interventions to address the problem. New York State and its local governments subsidize the majority of methadone maintenance treatment programs and have few restrictions on dosing or duration of treatment.

It was in New York City that the pioneering research of Dole and Nyswander (see, e.g., Dole and Nyswander, 1965) established methadone maintenance as a legitimate pharmacotherapy for opiate addiction in the mid-1960s. New York's practitioners probably accept to a larger extent than those in other states the proposition that relatively high doses of methadone are required to provide a blockade against the euphoria provided by heroin. Methadone providers in New York tend to subscribe to a blockade model of maintenance, in which the methadone dose is increased until it prevents withdrawal symptoms for a full 24-hour period, rather than being limited to a preset maximum dose. Finally, in New York, detoxification is viewed as a short-term intervention, typically necessary where there are medical complications or mixed addictions present. In general, it is seen there as an adjunct to treatment and is not regarded as a desirable or reasonable alternative to long-term methadone maintenance.

California did not establish methadone maintenance programs until the early 1970s. The first state oversight agency, the Research Advisory Panel (RAP), viewed methadone as appropriate for detoxification but regarded methadone maintenance as a "treatment of last resort." This view continued under the Department of Alcohol and Drug Programs, which assumed administrative responsibility later in the 1970s, and led to an emphasis during the 1980s on low-dose treatment of limited duration. The majority of methadone providers in California during the 1970s and 1980s maintained average dose levels of around 40 mg, a level considerably under the 60 mg average recommended by NIDA. More recently, state dosing policies have changed, so that by early 1994, only 18 perecent of patients received a dose under 40 mg, some 28 percent received doses between 40 and 59 mg, about 45 percent received doses between 60 and 80 mg, and about 8 percent were on doses greater than 80 mg.

Independently, as local government budgets were constrained in 1976 and thereafter as a result of Proposition 13, many California counties began to withdraw their subsidy of methadone maintenance treatment programs. By the mid-1980s, the majority of methadone treatment funds were provided out-of-pocket by clients' fees (see chapter 6). However, for several years California has subsidized methadone treatment for addicted women who are pregnant or postpartum, for addicts who are HIV-positive patients, and for certain other specified groups of addicts.

The results of these state policies are evident in the data discussed above and highlighted in Table 3-3. First, many more opiate addicts receive methadone maintenance in New York than in California. Second, the California emphasis on subsidized treatment for pregnant and postpartum addicts has resulted in women making up 43 percent of the January 1, 1992, patient census in that state, compared to only 34 percent of the census in New York State. Finally, a comparison of the censuses for January 1, 1992, and January 1, 1993, indicates that while New York increased methadone treatment slots by 6 percent, California increased its slots by about 1 percent. Furthermore, the turnover of maintenance slots in California (number of discharges in 1992 divided by the January 1, 1992 census) is more than twice that of New York, even when discharge numbers are reduced by removing "satisfactory discharges" and inter-program transfers.

TABLE 3-3 California and New York Methadone Maintenance Patient Flow in 1992

| | California | | | | | | New York | | | | | |
| | Males | | Females | | Total | | Males | | Females | | Total | |
	N	%	N	%	N	%	N	%	N	%	N	%
January 1992 Census	9,024	56.8	6,872	43.2	15,896	100	26,088	66.3	13,252	33.7	39,340	100
Admissions	7,592	57.0	5,936	43.0	13,328	100	9,657	68.7	4,400	31.3	14,057	100
All Discharges	6,822	57.0	5,139	43.0	11,961	100	8,007	68.7	3,642	31.3	11,649	100
January 1993 Census	9,095	56.6	6,988	43.4	16,083	100	27,692	66.4	13,987	33.6	41,679	100
Growth	71	0.8	116	1.7	187	1.2	1,604	6.2	735	5.6	2,339	6.0
Uncorrected Turnover	—	75.0	—	73.5	—	74.4	—	30.7	—	27.5	—	29.6
Satisfactory discharge	510	7.5	437	8.5	947	7.9	541	6.8	250	6.9	791	6.8
Transferred	716	10.5	862	16.8	1,578	13.2	946	11.8	552	15.2	1,498	12.9
Turnover		67.7		62.2		65.3		.271		.233		.258
Turnover		62.0		55.9		59.4		.250		.214		.238

SOURCES: California Department of Alcohol and Drug Programs; New York State Office of Alcoholism and Substance Abuse Services.

Although New York and California, respectively, treat the largest number of opiate addicts, they differ in the number of patients served, the number of women in treatment, the type of treatment provided and subsidized, and dosing policies. These differences are due to individual state philosophies, policies, and regulations, which are also reflected in general differences in public subsidies. These state differences suggest a useful research opportunity to study the consequences of alternative financing and regulatory approaches to methadone maintenance, the results of which could inform the drafting of new regulations or clinical practice guidelines.

SUMMARY

This chapter presents data that show that heroin use occurs, along a continuum including those who have ever used opiates, those who ever become dependent on opiates, those who become addicted, and those who are treated for addiction. However, no effort has been made to estimate the size of the heroin addict population, even though this figure is of great interest to policymakers.

There is considerable uncertainty about the size of the heroin addict population. Almost all analysts believe the total number of heroin addicts to be at least 500,000, though estimates that range up to one million are sometimes mentioned. A committee of the National Research Council (NRC) in 1989 analyzed the estimates of the prevalence of intravenous drug use (IVDU), which is dominated by heroin use. B.D. Spencer, who was asked by the NRC committee to evaluate the accuracy of the IVDU estimates, concluded: "The accuracy of the estimates of the number of [users] is not objectively ascertainable, but the estimate (of about 1 million) could well be off by a factor of 2; that is, the true number could conceivably be smaller than 500,000 or greater than 2 million. The closeness of several of the estimates is not persuasive because they cannot be regarded as independent estimates" (Spencer, 1989).

Reuter (1993) reviewed the literature regarding the prevalence of heroin addiction and concluded: "Since the HPI [Heroin Problems Index]-based estimate in 1981, there has been only one formal estimate of the number of heroin addicts nationally (Cooley et al. 1990), which used DAWN's [Drug Abuse Waring Network's] heroin-related ER mentions to produce a figure of 853,000 for 1987. This number, developed by an adaptation of the HPI technique, has not acquired much authority; the sensitivity to highly uncertain anchor city estimates is probably the primary reason."

Gerstein and Harwood (1990) estimated the population of all drug users clearly in need of treatment at 1.5 million. They did not make a separate estimate of heroin addicts in need of treatment.

The lower range of the estimates of the total addict population does not appear to be in question. The figure is high enough to make the point that the estimated 115,000 methadone patients in maintenance treatment is modest relative to the size of the addict population.[3]

REFERENCES

Anglin, MD, and McGlothlin, WH. 1985. Methadone maintenance in California: A decade's experience. In: L. Brill and C. Winick (eds.), *The Yearbook of Substance Use and Abuse.* Vol. 3. New York: Human Sciences Press.

Anthony, JC, Warner, LA, and Kessler, RC. 1994. Comparative epidemiology of dependence of tobacco, alcohol, controlled substances, and inhalants: Basic findings from the National Comorbidity Study. *Clinical and Experimental Psychopharmacology.* (in press.)

Anthony, JC, and Helzer, JE. 1991. Syndromes of drug abuse and dependence. In: L. N. Robins and D. A. Regier (eds.), *Psychiatric Disorder in America.* New York: The Free Press.

Ball, JC and Greberman, SB. 1994. Lifetime arrest rates of heroin addicts in Baltimore. In: *Problems of Drug Dependence, 1993: Proceedings of the 55th Annual Scientific Meeting of the College on Problems of Drug Dependence,* L.S. Harris, ed., Vol. 2: Abstracts. NIDA Research Monograph 141, Rockville, Md. P. 42.

Ball, JC, and Ross, A. 1991. *The Effectiveness of Methadone Maintenance Treatment: Patients, Programs, Services, and Outcomes.* New York: Springer-Verlag.

Biernacki, P. 1986. *Pathways from Heroin Addiction: Recovery Without Treatment.* Philadelphia: Temple University Press.

Courtwright, DT. 1982. *Dark Paradise: Opiate Addiction in America Before 1940.* Cambridge, Mass.: Harvard University Press.

Dole, VP, and Nyswander, M. 1965. A medical treatment for diacetylmorphine (heroin) addiction. *Journal of the American Medical Association.* 193:80–84.

Fiorentine, R, and Anglin, MD. 1993. Perceiving need for drug treatment: A look at eight hypotheses. Unpublished manuscript. Los Angeles: University of California, Drug Abuse Research Center.

---

[3]It should be noted that the incarcerated population includes a considerable number of heroin addicts who are unable to participate in methadone treatment programs.

Flynn, PM, Craddock, S, Gail, MS, Luckey, JW, and Hubbard, RL. 1994. *Client Characteristics Among Admissions to Methadone Treatment Programs in Two National Samples: 1979–981, 1991–993*. Research Triangle Park, NC.

General Accounting Office. 1990. *Methadone Maintenance: Some Treatment Programs Are Not Effective; Greater Federal Oversight Needed*. GAO/HRD-90-104. Washington, D.C.: U.S. Government Printing Office.

Gerstein, Dr, and Harwood, HJ (eds.). 1990. *Treating Drug Problems*. Vol. I Washington, D.C.: National Academy Press.

Hser, Y, Anglin, MD, and Powers, K. 1993. A 24 year follow-up of California narcotics addicts. *Archives of General Psychiatry* 50:577–584.

Johnston, LD, O'Malley, PM, and Bachman, JG. 1993. *National Survey Results on Drug Use from the Monitoring the Future Study, 1975–1992*. Vol. 2 *College Students and Young Adults*. Rockville, Md. National Institute on Drug Abuse.

Musto, DF. 1973, 1987. *The American Disease: Origins of Narcotic Control*. New York: Oxford University Press.

National Institute on Alcohol Abuse and Alcoholism. 1994. *Eighth Special Report to the U.S. Congress on Alcohol and Health*. NIH Publication No. 94-3699. Rockville, Md. NIAA, DHHS.

O'Donnel, JA, Voss, HL, Clayton, RR, Slatin, GT, and Room, R. 1976. *Young Men and Drugs: A Nationwide Survey*. NIDA Research Monograph 5, DHEW Publication No. (ADM) 76-311, Washington, D.C.

Reuter, P. 1993. Prevalence estimation and policy formulation. *Journal of Drug Issues* 23(2):167–184.

Rhodes, P. 1993. Synthetic estimation applied to the prevalence of drug use. *Journal of Drug Issues* 23(2):297–322.

Rittenhouse, JD. 1977. *The Epidemiology of Heroin and Other Narcotics*. NIDA Research Monograph 16, Rockville, Md.

Robins, LN. 1974. *The Vietnam Drug User Returns*. Special Action Office Monograph, Series A, No. 2. Washington, D.C.: U.S. Government Printing Office.

Robins, LN, and Murphy, GE. 1967. Drug use in a normal population of young Negro men. *American Journal of Public Health* 57:1580–1596.

Simpson, DD, Joe, GW, Lehman, WEK, and Sells, SB. 1986. Addiction careers: Etiology, treatment, and 12-year follow-up procedures. *Journal of Drug Issues* 16:107–121.

Simpson, DD, and Savage, LJ. 1980. Treatment re-entry and outcomes of opioid addicts during a four-year follow-up after drug abuse treatment in the United States. *Bulletin on Narcotics* 32(4):1–10.

Spencer, BD. 1989. On the accuracy of estimates of numbers of intravenous drug users. In *AIDS: Sexual Behavior and Intravenous Drug Use*. Washington, D.C.: National Research Council.

Vaillant, GE. 1973. A 20-year follow-up of New York narcotic addicts. *Archives of General Psychiatry* 29:237–241.

4

Methadone Diversion Control

The concern for methadone diversion preceded the issuance of FDA methadone regulations in 1972, influenced the views of policymakers writing the regulations, and continues to shape the regulations today as thoroughly as does a concern for the medical use of methadone to treat opiate addiction.

The legitimate public interest in the control of methadone diversion stems from methadone's status as a schedule II controlled substance and the fact that it is a long-acting opiate, itself addictive, having a potential for abuse both by opiate addicts and by nonaddicts. Under certain circumstances, methadone, like any other opiate, can be dangerous and life-threatening. An examination of relevant data, however, indicates that the actual level of abuse and harm from illicit methadone falls short of its hypothetical potential for abuse.

The purpose of this chapter is to examine the degree to which methadone diversion is a public safety and public health problem within the context of federal methadone regulations. The discussion addresses the following topics:the early concern over diversion and its impact on the development of methadone regulations and legislation, official views on methadone diversion, the available data on diversion, the methods of methadone diversion, the characteristics and motivations of users of street methadone, the public safety and health consequences of diversion, and conclusions and recommendations.

EARLY CONCERN OVER DIVERSION

The concept of opiate substitution therapy using methadone in the treatment of opiate dependence was a radical break with the established approach to narcotics control in the United States, an approach that had been enforced by the Federal Bureau of Narcotics (FBN) since the 1920s (Courtwright, 1992; Musto, 1987). A prior attempt at treating opiate addiction by morphine had been established by some cities around 1920. This had been vigorously resisted by law enforcement agencies, resulting in the closure of these clinics. The FBN upheld this antimaintenance position for the next 40 years. The use of methadone to treat opiate addiction thus violated the FBN's long-standing policy against maintenance treatment of addiction.

The experimental work of Drs. Vincent Dole and Marie Nyswander on methadone maintenance at the Rockefeller Institute in New York City in the early 1960s led to an initial report on methadone treatment in the *Journal of the American Medical Association* (Dole and Nyswander, 1965). Following the success of the studies on methadone by Dole and his colleagues, the number of methadone treatment programs began to increase in all major U.S. cities. In 1968, fewer than 400 patients were enrolled in methadone maintenance programs nationwide. By January 1973, the number of patients enrolled in federal and nonfederal maintenance programs had increased to 73,000 (U.S. Congress, 1973c, p. 4). Administration of some of these programs was lax, resulting in the diversion of methadone to the street market by various means. In addition, in the early 1970s, a number of cities, particularly those on the East Coast, experienced a decline in heroin supplies, owing to a combination of enforcement efforts and dock strikes; the relative scarcity of heroin stimulated the market demand for illicit methadone as a substitute for heroin. The Bureau of Narcotics and Dangerous Drugs (BNDD, successor to the FBN, FDA, and the Special Action Office for Drug Abuse Prevention developed regulations for the operation of methadone programs primarily in order to control the problem of diversion.[1]

The concerns over methadone diversion of the early 1970s shaped many of the provisions of FDA methadone regulations issued in December 1972. Although it is not always clear whether a specific provision was designed to prevent diversion or to serve some other purpose or both, the following provisions are among the main ones that seem to have been included primarily to limit the likelihood that methadone would reach the street:

• Requiring that methadone in the treatment of opiate addiction be dispensed only by programs licensed by the federal government;
• Placing limits on the dispensing of methadone for treatment of narcotic addiction in hospitals;

---

[1] A number of newspaper articles published at the time contributed to the view that methadone diversion was a problem. The tone of the articles is suggested by some of their titles: "Study finds black market developing in methadone" (*New York Times*, January 2, 1972, by J.W. Markham); "Curse or cure? Controversy balloons over use of methadone as a heroin substitute" (*Wall Street Journal*, July 27, 1972, by I. Walters); "Methadone: Will it spread addiction?" (*National Observer*, May 29, 1972, by A. Gribbon).

- Requiring that patients be enrolled in only one program;
- Requiring physician justification in patient records for daily dosages greater than 100 mg;
- Specifying strict timetables and criteria for granting (and rescinding) take-home doses to patients;
- Denying take-home privileges to patients receiving a daily dose greater than 100 mg.

The requirement for providing counseling and rehabilitative services to patients, while mainly concerned with treatment goals, could also be construed in terms of diversion prevention on the grounds that rehabilitated methadone patients would be less likely to use their medication irresponsibly, nor would they have reason to do so if, as a result of counseling and other treatment, they had quit using other illicit drugs and had become involved in school or work.

In a series of Senate and House hearings held in 1972 and 1973 on the various bills that later become the Narcotic Addict Treatment Act of 1974, BNDD presented its views on methadone diversion. In their testimony, BNDD officials relied on a number of sources to document their position that diversion was a serious problem (see U.S. Congress, 1973a, pp. 657–663; U.S. Congress, 1973b, pp. 18–36, 53–57). BNDD officials cited research studies that had been conducted on diversion. One of the main studies referred to was by Chambers and Inciardi (1972), an interview study of 95 active heroin addicts in New York City in 1971. Eighty-seven percent of these addicts reported that they had been offered the opportunity to purchase illicit methadone at least once in the past six months; 55 percent had actually purchased diverted methadone during this period. Thirteen percent had sold methadone illegally at some time, 8 percent in the prior six months.[2]

BNDD also presented the results of a number of undercover operations in various cities that involved illegal and excessive dispensing by physicians in private practice or associated with treatment programs.[3] A further indication of the extent of methadone diversion, according to BNDD, was an increase in arrests in various cities involving the sale or possession of illegal methadone.

---

[2] Other research studies on methadone diversion and related subjects (e.g., primary methadone addiction) conducted in the early 1970s include Chambers and Bergen (1973), Sapira et al. (1973), Stephens and Weppner (1973a, 1973b), Walter et al (1973), Weppner and Stephens (1973), and Weppner et al (1972).

[3] The most famous of these was that of Dr. Thomas W. Moore, Jr., of Washington, D.C., who dispensed methadone to several hundred patients who paid from $15 for 50 tablets to $75 for 200 tablets each week. He was eventually convicted on 22 counts of illegally dispensing or prescribing under the Controlled Substances Act of 1970 in a case that went to the Supreme Court (U.S. v. Moore, 423 U.S. 122 (1975)).

Another source of data on methadone diversion offered by BNDD was deaths attributed to methadone. From 1970 through the first six months of 1972, the percentage of drug-related deaths attributed to methadone by medical examiners increased from 6 percent to 25 percent in New York City and from 20 percent to 40 percent in Washington, D.C.[4] (This increase parallels the rapid increase in the number of methadone programs and patients during this period, as well as the shortage of heroin supplies that resulted in a decline in heroin-related deaths.)

In June 1972, BNDD established a more systematic program for documenting the relative frequency of abuse of controlled substances. The Drug Abuse Warning Network (DAWN) collected data on drug "mentions" from a variety of sources, including hospital emergency rooms and inpatient facilities, student health centers, county medical examiners and coroners, and community drug crisis centers; later, DAWN reports were limited to hospital emergency rooms and medical examiners. (Briefly, "mentions" refer to medical examiner report that a descendent tested positive for a particular substance. A detailed discussion of drug mentions, "methadone-related death," and of the problems in interpreting DAWN data is presented below.)

As shown in Table 4-1, results from the early months of the operation of DAWN indicated that as heroin reports were declining, methadone reports were increasing. BNDD interpreted this as an increase in the availability of diverted methadone.

BNDD identified four main sources of methadone diversion: (1) the activities of "unscrupulous practitioners" who "wrote script" (i.e., prescriptions) for methadone; (2) the negligent operation of legitimate programs that resulted in unaccounted-for shortages of methadone stocks; (3) the diversion by patients enrolled in methadone programs; and (4) robberies from methadone clinics and pharmacies and hijackings from trucks transporting methadone. Of these four, the most important were the script-writing practitioners and sale by methadone patients.

---

[4] References in this chapter to medical examiner data pertain to data about drug-related deaths.

TABLE 4-1 DAWN Reports of Heroin and Methadone September 1972–January 1973

	Heroin		Methadone	
	No. of reports	%	No. of reports	%
September	643	85.5	93	14.5
October	683	76.7	159	23.3
November	667	64.6	236	35.4
December	552	62.1	209	37.9
January	680	65	235	35

NOTE: DAWN = Drug Abuse Warning Network. Data are based on 64 reporting facilities in 38 Standard Metropolitan Statistical Areas. Figures from the initial DAWN system did not differentiate between reports of drug-related deaths and reports of other drug-related incidents.

THE NARCOTIC ADDICT TREATMENT ACT OF 1974

The Narcotic Addict Treatment Act (NATA) addressed the two main sources of methadone diversion, namely, practitioners and patients. First, the act required that practitioners who wished to dispense narcotics drugs for maintenance treatment or detoxification needed to obtain a separate registration from the Attorney General; it also specified that such registration could be suspended for failure to comply with the treatment standards established by the Secretary of Health, Education, and Welfare (now Health and Human Services) and the security standards established by the Attorney General. Practitioners who continued to dispense narcotic drugs for maintenance or detoxification without a registration could be prosecuted under provisions of the Controlled Substances Act. Second, the potential for diversion by patients was addressed in the section that required the Secretary to establish standards (after consultation with the Attorney General) for the amount of methadone that could be provided to patients for unsupervised use (i.e., take homes).

The NATA created a closed distribution system, in which only approved programs could purchase methadone for treatment. This new system effectively put out of business the doctors who had been prescribing methadone indiscriminately, without regard for treatment. The impact of the NATA, combined with that of the FDA regulations of December 1972, which became effective in March 1973, on the availability of street methadone is less clear. According to DEA officials, the passage of the NATA in 1974 and the inspection activities of DEA to ensure compliance by methadone programs resulted in a decline in methadone diversion, as indicated by reductions in methadone mentions in emergency room episodes and by medical examiners (U.S. Congress, 1989, pp. 138–139). Methadone mentions by medical examiners reporting to DAWN declined from a three-month moving average of 88 mentions in August 1974 to 47 in July 1976. Over this same period, methadone mentions declined from 11.1 percent to 6.6 percent of all drug mentions (National Institute on Drug Abuse, 1977). The U.S. General Accounting Office (1976) also reported that, based on data from DEA and local police departments, illicit sales of methadone were declining and that what sales did occur consisted of small quantities of take-home doses.

By contrast, two NIDA-funded studies on methadone diversion conducted by Fordham University in 1972–1973 and 1974–1975 indicated that the *short-term* impact of the NATA and FDA's restrictive take-home policy on the availability of diverted methadone was minimal (Martin et al.,; Martin et al., 1975, summarized in Inciardi, 1977). The Fordham studies found that illicit methadone was readily available on the streets of all cities investigated both before and after enactment of NATA. In fact, data from New York and Philadelphia suggested that the use of illicit methadone had become more widespread in the latter period.

Despite its availability, only 4 percent of the street addicts interviewed the second study said that methadone was the main drug they used. The primary reason for the use of illicit methadone was for self-treatment of addiction ("to keep from getting sick"). Only a minority of respondents reported that they used the drug "to get high." (See chapter 2 for a discussion of the methadone "high.") The studies did find that law enforcement officials, at both federal and local levels, placed a low priority on diverted methadone relative to their enforcement efforts against other illicit drugs.

MORE RECENT OFFICIAL VIEWS ON DIVERSION

House Select Committee Hearings

Methadone diversion has continued to occupy the attention of DEA (successor to BNDD and members of Congress, particularly the House Select Committee on Narcotics Abuse and Control. At committee hearings, testimony focused on the seriousness of the diversion problem, with only isolated voices of dissent (U.S. Congress, 1978, 1989, 1990). A report of the Select Committee in 1978 concluded:

From a public health perspective, methadone diversion and illicit use represent a significant threat. This committee documented numerous cases of primary methadone addiction, of drug death due to illicit methadone and of emergency episodes involving methadone. Illicit methadone must be minimized; that is why the committee has concluded that take-home dosage units represent a major threat. The benefits of methadone treatment are great but the social and public health costs of its widespread use are also great [U.S. Congress, 1978, p. 29].

At a hearing on August 2, 1989, the Select Committee heard from DEA officials regarding a month-long DEA undercover investigation of methadone diversion in the vicinity of methadone treatment programs in the five boroughs of New York City in August 1988, during which agents were able to purchase 98 containers totaling 5.45 grams of methadone, with an average price of about $35 per 80 mg (U.S. Congress, 1989, pp. 150–152; A.L. Carter, DEA, personal communication, April 15, 1994). Agents observed as many as 20 to 25 people selling their methadone at a given location. As a result of this investigation, DEA, in cooperation with FDA and the New York State Bureau of Controlled Substances, inspected five programs near which illegal methadone sales had been observed. The violations found at two of these programs led to the initiation of proceedings to have their DEA registration revoked (the cited problems were later corrected). The results of this action appeared on a nationwide news broadcast and were reported at a hearing of the Select Committee in March 1990 (U.S. Congress, 1990). Thus, methadone diversion remained before members of Congress and the public.

Perspective of the Drug Enforcement Administration

The Drug Enforcement Administration has responsibility, under the Controlled Substances Act of 1970 and the Narcotic Addict Treatment Act of 1974, for preventing the diversion and abuse of methadone by establishing and monitoring security and record-keeping procedures for licensed methadone programs. DEA continues to maintain BNDD's earlier concern over the potential for methadone diversion. In DEA's view, "Methadone is an addictive, euphoria-producing drug with a high street value, and we believe it obvious that the dispensing of such a drug to an addict population, which by definition has shown itself to be more likely to abuse drugs than the general population, should be done only within a tightly regulated framework" (U.S. Congress, 1989, p. 134).

In addition to the fact that the sale of methadone is illegal, DEA regards diverted methadone as the source of other public health and safety problems, mainly as a cause or contributor to drug-related deaths, as a way for heroin addicts to manage their habit without entering treatment, as a source of income to support the use of other illicit drugs, and as a means of primary methadone addiction.

In DEA's view, record-keeping and security procedures have effectively limited methadone diversion at the manufacturing, distribution, and program levels. Most of the diversion now seen, DEA asserts, occurs as a result of poor adherence to treatment standards, which allows patients to sell methadone on the streets. From DEA's perspective, lax program administration is evidenced by a variety of factors, including a trend toward increasing the number of patients at the expense of comprehensive services, a reluctance by programs to rescind take-home privileges following drug tests that are positive for drugs or negative for methadone, a movement toward higher daily methadone doses, indefinite maintenance program policies, and poor control over enrollment in multiple programs. DEA is also concerned about trends toward nonmedical administration, the increasing appearance of privately run "for profit" programs, the emergence of programs in areas with low historic problems with heroin use (e.g., rural southeastern states), and budget cutbacks that have negatively affected publicly funded programs.

All of these factors, in DEA's judgment, potentially increase the opportunity for patients to sell methadone on the street. DEA testimony before congressional committees and interviews of DEA officials by IOM committee members indicate that DEA appears to favor policies that would provide for comprehensive services, further tighten up treatment regulations (especially as regards take home practices), and improve program monitoring to ensure compliance with regulations (again, especially as regards take home doses).

DEA officials often note that many methadone patients are polydrug users and that they continue to use drugs as evidenced by urine tests. At first sight, this observation may seem beside the point since methadone is specific only to opiate addiction. But the observation becomes relevant to DEA's perspective on diversion in regard to two points. First, DEA (like its predecessor, BNDD) has strongly argued that methadone treatment, in addition to dispensing the medication, must include comprehensive medical and social services, which should include addressing other drug use. Second, and more pertinent to diversion, methadone patients who continue to use other illicit drugs have an incentive to sell their methadone to purchase other drugs; thus, in DEA's view, methadone programs that fail to address other drug use may, in effect, be subsidizing drug abuse.

According to Eugene Haislip, Deputy Assistant Administrator for Diversion Control of DEA, the failure by programs to address other drug use creates "little incentive for an individual to become drug free because their steady supply of methadone provides them with a constant source of illicit income with which to purchase other drugs, primarily cocaine. Any broadening of present standards regarding take-home dosages of methadone can only be expected to exacerbate the problem" (see U.S. Congress, 1989, p. 136).

THE DATA ON DIVERSION

All of the problems cited by DEA that are associated with methadone diversion have occurred and will continue to occur to some extent so long as methadone programs exist. However, in assessing the degree of seriousness of methadone diversion as a public safety and public health problem (and therefore as a problem in need of a certain level of intervention), it is not enough to document instances of harm. What is needed is to determine (within the constraints of available data and methodology) how often methadone diversion and related consequences occur, how harmful they are, and how methadone diversion compares with the diversion of other drugs. This section offers information from a variety of data sources as a preliminary answer to that question.

Drug Abuse Warning Network Data

One of the main sources relied upon by DEA to document the extent of diversion is the methadone "mentions" in the Drug Abuse Warning Network (DAWN). Specifically, DAWN data consist of reports of "methadone-related deaths" from medical examiners. In addition to "mentions" however, DAWN data also include other emergency room data. A discussion of methadone toxicity and toxicology will help place the following discussion of DAWN and methadone-related deaths in context (see Barrett et al., 1993; Gottschalk et al., 1977; Karch, 1993).

With typical maintenance dosing, methadone has a half-life of about 24 hours. As with all opiates, toxicity is thought to be the result of respiratory depression due to decreased sensitivity of the brain's respiratory center to the stimulatory effect of carbon dioxide. There is, however, no clear definition of what constitutes a toxic or fatal blood methadone level. One reason for the difficulty of determining a toxic blood methadone level is drug interaction. A given blood methadone level may or may not be toxic depending on the presence of other drugs, which may augment or counteract any toxic effects of methadone.

Another factor that complicates establishing a toxic methadone level is individual variability in susceptibility to methadone's effects. Opiate tolerance is a major determinant of this variability. As opiate users develop tolerance, they need progressively higher doses to achieve the desired effect. The rate at which tolerance develops depends in part on the pattern of use. Some patients who are highly tolerant to methadone suffer no toxic effects at blood methadone levels that would be toxic to a person lacking tolerance.

Therefore, because of the phenomena of drug interactions and tolerance, considerable overlap exists between therapeutic and toxic blood methadone levels. One cannot rely solely on blood methadone levels to determine if methadone toxicity is the cause of death. The main implication of this discussion is that existing medical examiner data, as reflected in DAWN, most likely overcount the number of drug-related deaths in DAWN reporting cities that can be attributed solely to methadone or to which methadone would be contributing.

The difficulty in accurately interpreting DAWN medical examiner data is highlighted by two surveys conducted by Gottschalk and his colleagues (Gottschalk et al., 1979; Gottschalk and Cravey, 1980) of psychoactive drug-involved deaths in medical examiner and coroner offices in nine large cities. The first survey reviewed 2,000 deaths that occurred between 1972 and 1974; the second examined 1,004 deaths that occurred during the first eight months of 1975. Both surveys showed clearly defined differences in toxicological findings between different cities. In the second survey, for instance, methadone was detected in 52 percent of the cases reported in New York—more than three times the percentage of the next highest city. Wide intercity differences were also found in the rank order of drugs as to the cause of death. In New York, methadone was ranked as the primary cause of death in 47 percent of all cases. In other reporting centers, the percentage ranged from 0 percent to 11 percent.

In attempting to account for these disparities, Gottschalk and his colleagues found significant differences in the toxicological examinations performed by laboratories at different regional offices. Moreover, they found that even when the toxicological results were the same in different offices, the interpretation of those results often differed. The investigators concluded that intercity differences in methadone-detected deaths were "largely artifactual and not true differences representative of epidemiological characteristics. Rather, these differences are representative of instrumental or methodological sophistication and/or personal or departmental emphasis. Until these interlaboratory differences can be further delineated and corrected, the epidemiological characteristics of psychoactive drug-involved deaths must be cautiously interpreted" (Gottschalk and Cravey, 1980, p. 56).

A final point regarding methadone-involved deaths. The number of decedents who have methadone in their body is a direct function of the number of people who are enrolled in methadone treatment. As the number of methadone patients increases, so will the number of deaths in which methadone is detected. If all heroin addicts were enrolled in methadone and other types of treatment programs and if these treatment programs were successful in greatly reducing, if not eliminating, heroin use, then long-acting methadone would be detected in virtually all deaths involving opiates (Wright, 1992). This is why any sophisticated analysis of methadone's involvement in drug-related deaths (or in emergency room mentions) should include the treatment status of the decedent. Unfortunately, such information is not usually available.

Harris County, Texas

An opportunity to look behind the meaning of the oft-used term "methadone-related death" was afforded by a series of drug-related deaths in Harris County, Texas, in 1991. These deaths were widely publicized in the *Houston Chronicle* at the time and, on February 21, 1993, received nation-wide television attention on the CBS News program "60 Minutes." The Centers for Disease Control (CDC) was asked to investigate (for the background to the CDC investigation, see the chapter appendix). The CDC investigators restricted themselves to examining the Harris County medical examiner cases on decedents who tested positive for methadone on postmortem drug testing (methadone-detected deaths) from January 1, 1987, through December 31, 1992. They analyzed data from four sources: Harris County medical examiner data, methadone maintenance treatment data, review by three independent pathologists, and DAWN medical examiner data.

Harris County Medical Examiner Data

The investigators examined autopsy data on the 91 methadone-detected cases seen by the Harris County medical examiner from 1987 through 1992, of which 27 occurred in 1991. Cases were grouped by cause of death: toxicity, natural, and trauma. Of the 91 decedents, the CDC investigators found polydrug toxicity to be the most frequent primary cause of death, accounting for 37 percent of the deaths. The second most frequently cited cause was methadone toxicity, accounting for 12 percent. (In all, toxicity accounted for 59 percent of deaths; natural causes, 22 percent; and trauma, 19 percent). In addition, they found that the increase in methadone-detected deaths in 1990 and 1991 in Harris County reflected an increase in deaths due to polydrug use, rather than an increase in the frequency of methadone use alone.

Methadone Maintenance Treatment Data

In order to determine which of the methadone-detected decedents had legally obtained methadone, the investigators collected information regarding the decedents' history of methadone maintenance treatment. They relied on the 18 methadone maintenance treatment programs then operating in Harris County to supply treatment information on the methadone-detected decedents. Of the 91 methadone-detected decedents, 31 (34 percent) were identified as having ever been enrolled in one or more of the programs, while 60 (66 percent) had no documented history of enrollment.[7] Of the 31 decedents who had a history of methadone treatment, 18 were enrolled in methadone maintenance at the time of death. Thus, the majority (80 percent) of methadone-detected decedents were not enrolled in a Harris Country methadone maintenance program at the time of death, suggesting that they probably obtained methadone from other sources. These other sources could have included inpatient detoxification programs, retail pharmacies, or cancer treatment facilities, as well as methadone diverted to the street.

Independent Pathologists' Review

The 27 Harris County medical examiner methadone-detected cases for 1991 were reviewed by three independent, out-of-state forensic pathologists. These 27 deaths were grouped into three causal categories: "primary cause," "contributing cause," and "unrelated." Two of the three reviewers agreed that methadone was the primary cause of death in 3 cases (11 percent), the contributing cause in 9 cases (35 percent), and unrelated to death in 14 cases (54 percent); the three were unanimous that methadone was the primary cause of death in one case. (The three pathologists did not meet face-to-face; they exercised their judgment about probable cause of death without the benefit of agreed-upon a priori criteria; nor did they review the bases for their agreements and disagreements after the fact.)

Drug Abuse Warning Network (DAWN) Medical Examiner Data

The CDC researchers drew on DAWN data to investigate trends in methadone and heroin/morphine mentions in reports of drug-abuse deaths from

---

[7] Some of these 60 decedents might have been enrolled in one of three clinics that were closed in March and April 1992, whose records were not available to CDC investigators. These decedents might also have been enrolled in programs outside Harris County.

1980 to 1991 in 55 urban county medical examiner offices in 20 states. The investigators found no evidence of a general increase in the prevalence of methadone use among people dying from drug-related causes. They did find, however, that the number of heroin mentions increased almost threefold.

The CDC investigation revealed that although the number of methadone-detected deaths in Harris County, Texas, had increased in 1990 and 1991, deaths attributable to methadone toxicity alone did not increase. Multiple drugs or alcohol were found in 85 percent of the methadone-detected decedents. Although methadone by itself may not have caused these deaths, methadone in combination with other substances (particularly other respiratory depressants) *may* have contributed to death. Without knowing the decedents' tolerance to methadone and other opiates, and without reliable information about decedents' methadone maintenance treatment histories, it was not possible for the CDC investigators to determine what role methadone had played in the death.

In summary, the CDC investigation found that the number of reported methadone-detected deaths in Harris County increased in 1990 and 1991, but deaths definitively explained by methadone toxicity did not increase. Rather, the increase was only in polydrug deaths in which methadone was one of two or more drugs.

Other Data on Diversion

DEA cites DAWN data in support of its view that a significant amount of the available methadone produced each year is diverted and that street methadone is a major drug of abuse. In a table prepared by DEA using 1991 DAWN data, methadone ranked twentieth out of the top 20 controlled substances in terms of drug mentions at hospital emergency rooms. Twenty-six hundred (2,680) events involving methadone produced this ranking, virtually the same as in the previous three years. Above methadone in the list were cocaine (102,727 mentions), marijuana (15,182), diazepam (14,851), methamphetamine (4,981), and LSD (3,912). If the number of DAWN mentions is regarded as a measure of abuse, it is difficult to argue from the above figures alone that methadone is a *major* drug of abuse. Furthermore, these figures do not exclude methadone mentions for people enrolled in methadone programs who may be seen in emergency rooms for a variety of presenting conditions having little or nothing to do with their use of methadone. [8]

Another argument that DEA puts forward about the dangers of methadone diversion is based on the ratio of the methadone-related deaths, as reported to DAWN by medical examiners, to the amount of methadone produced and distributed annually. Haislip, in a 1991 speech in Boston to a plenary session of the National Methadone Conference, argued that heroin was only two to four times more lethal than methadone, depending on one's estimate of the kilograms of heroin available in the United States each year. He said:

> If you assume the smaller quantity of heroin is available [7,000 kilograms], . . . then heroin produces injuries about four times more often per kilogram than methadone. Well, that is a lot but remember that all the heroin is illegal, the methadone is all legal. If you assume the higher range [of heroin, i.e., 14,600 kilograms], . . . then it [heroin] is only twice as potent as methadone. . . . So you can see that this is the nature of our concern:a legitimate drug which causes injuries at such a level as to be comparable to an entirely illicit drug. (E. Haislip, National Methadone Conference, Boston, 1991.)

The detailed DEA argument is as follows. Each year, about 1,800 kg of methadone are distributed in the United States; a larger quantity may be authorized for production but held in inventory. Approximately 90 percent of this methadone distributed treatment programs, the rest to research or to pharmacies or hospitals for use in pain treatment. In 1991, DAWN reported 430 deaths in which methadone was detected in the decedent. Using these figures, DEA estimates one methadone related death for every 3.8 kg of methadone distributed. [9]

If it was true that one death was caused by every 3.8 kg of methadone distributed, that would be an extraordinarily high mortality rate, an order of magnitude higher than the rate for any prescription drug approved by FDA. The DEA argument implies a causal relationship between volume of methadone distributed and mortality, but DEA makes no serious analytical effort to assess whether this implied causality is genuine or spurious. In fact, as indicated above, there are serious reasons to doubt causality. The DEA

---

[8] In 1989, NIDA staff conducted a field investigation of emergency rooms in New York City. Interviews with ER staff at one of the major DAWN reporting hospitals indicated that overdoses from methadone alone were rare; methadone mentions most often occurred in patients enrolled in methadone maintenance treatment who were being seen in the emergency room for diseases or other effects associated with drug abuse (National Institute on Drug Abuse, 1989).

[9] The calculation is as follows: (1,800 kg)(.90) = 1,620 kg used in methadone treatment programs; divided by 430 deaths = 3.8 kg per death.

argument cannot be accepted at face value but requires a clinical assessment of whether the presence of methadone in decedents was causal, contributing, or independent. Absent such analysis, the "ratio" argument should not be used to justify opposition to methadone pharmacotherapy.

Further examination of the DAWN data show that the methadone-related deaths are concentrated in older age groups. If a great deal of methadone were reaching the street and causing frequent deaths among street users, one would expect a relatively larger number of methadone-related deaths among younger rather than among older age groups. But just the opposite pattern appears in the 1991 DAWN data. No mentions of methadone were made in decedents 25 years old and younger, but for the 26–34 year-old group, there were 128 mentions (6.25 percent of total mentions) and for the 35 and older age group, 284 mentions (7.60 percent). As noted in chapter 3, *treated* heroin addicts are generally in their 30s, but the untreated are considerably younger.

In summary, the DAWN data on emergency room mentions and medical examiner mentions provides some idea of the extent of methadone diversion and its consequences. The results suggest that many of those found to have methadone in their bodies at death are probably using it legally as medication. But even if *all* cases were instances of diversion, the role of illicit methadone would still be much smaller than that of other legal and illicit drugs monitored by DAWN. Nor is there evidence of an increase in its contribution in recent years.

Drug Use Forecasting Data

Data from the Drug Use Forecasting (DUF) program (also discussed in chapter 3) for 1992 are shown in Table 4-2. These data indicate that fewer than 5 percent of male booked arrestees reported having ever used street methadone in all but 4 of 23 cities where DUF is conducted (the exceptions were New York, 9.3 percent, Portland (Ore.), 6.2 percent, San Diego, 5.0 percent and Philadelphia, 5.2 percent). Similarly low levels of self-reported use were recorded in the previous three years. Street use of methadone by female booked arrestees was higher (in DUF, women tend to have higher rates of use for all drug categories than do males). For instance, in 1992, street methadone use was reported by 5 percent or fewer of female booked arrestees in all but 6 of the 21 cities that interviewed females (the exceptions being New York (Manhattan) 18 percent, Portland (Ore.), 13 percent, Philadelphia, 6.6 percent,

TABLE 4.2 Percentage of Booked Arrestees Reporting Use of Street Methadone in DUF Cities (1992)

Site	(Total N)	Ever Used M	Ever Used F	Use in Last 30 Days M	Use in Last 30 Days F	Use in Last 3 Days M	Use in Last 3 Days F	Ever Dependent M	Ever Dependent F	Now Dependent M	Now Dependent F
New York	(1,057)	9.3	18.0	3.3	5.9	2.3	3.0	1.1	2.0	0.8	0.7
Portland (Ore.)	(1,096)	6.2	13.3	0.6	2.5	0.4	1.1	0.1	1.4	0.0	0.0
San Diego	(1,294)	5.6	6.0	0.7	0.5	0.3	0.5	0.9	1.8	0.1	0.0
Philadelphia	(1,574)	5.2	6.6	0.8	0.9	0.4	0.2	1.2	0.9	0.1	0.4
Detroit	(1,423)	5.0	4.6	0.3	0.2	0.1	0.2	0.3	0.9	0.0	0.0
Indianapolis	(1,239)	5.0	3.2	0.1	0.0	0.1	0.0	0.6	0.0	0.2	0.0
Denver	(1,358)	4.6	5.5	0.5	0.7	0.3	0.2	0.4	1.0	0.2	0.0
Phoenix	(1,630)	4.4	4.9	0.4	0.5	0.1	0.2	0.1	0.5	0.0	0.2
Los Angeles	(2,134)	3.8	5.4	0.8	0.6	0.3	0.0	0.3		0.3	0.1
Omaha[a]	(871)	3.7		0.3		0.2		0.5		0.2	
San Antonio	(1,014)	3.7	3.6	0.7	0.3	0.4	0.3	0.1	0.3	0.1	0.0
Kansas City	(1,286)	3.3	4.9	0.2	0.8	0.1	0.5	0.6	0.8	0.2	0.5
Houston	(1,359)	2.7	0.5	0.1	0.0	0.0	0.0	0.0	0.0	0.0	0.0
St. Louis	(1,261)	2.7	1.8	0.5	0.3	0.2	0.0	0.2	0.3	0.1	0.3
Cleveland	(1,134)	2.6	2.2	0.1	0.0	0.0	0.0	0.0	0.3	0.0	0.0
San Jose	(1,394)	2.6	3.4	0.5	0.7	0.4	0.2	0.6	0.7	0.3	0.0
Dallas	(1,400)	2.3	2.2	0.3	0.0	0.1	0.0	0.0	0.0	0.0	0.0
Birmingham	(1,000)	2.1	1.7	0.3	0.0	0.1	0.0	0.4	0.0	0.1	0.0
Ft. Lauderdale	(1,224)	1.9	2.2	0.1	0.0	0.0	0.0	0.4	0.0	0.1	0.0
Atlanta	(1,472)	1.8	1.7	0.4	0.2	0.4	0.2	0.1	0.4	0.1	0.2
New Orleans	(1,342)	1.1	1.1	0.4	0.3	0.2	0.3	0.1	0.3	0.1	0.3
Washington	(1,215)	1.0	1.9	0.2	1.0	0.1	0.6	0.0	0.3	0.0	0.3
Chicago[a]	(901)	0.6		0.0		0.0		0.0	1.0	0.0	0.0

NOTE: DUF = Drug Use Forecasting Program; M = male; and F = female.
[a] Women arrestees were not interviewed in these cities.

13 percent, and San Diego, 6.0 percent, Denver, 5.5 percent, and Los Angeles, 5.4 percent).[10]

In 1992, use in the prior 30 days was highest in New York: 25 (3.3 percent) male arrestees and 18 (5.9 percent) of female arrestees. Of the 25 male arrestees who had used street methadone in the prior 30 days, 44 percent had used it on three or fewer days. In cities other than New York, fewer than 1 percent of arrestees, both men and women, had used illegal methadone in the prior 30 days (except in Washington, DC, where the figure for women was just 1.0 percent). Reported dependence on street methadone was equally low; 2 percent of women arrestees and 1.1 percent of male arrestees in New York reported having ever being dependent on it. In all DUF cities and among both men and women, *current* dependence on street methadone was reported to be less than 1 percent.

Arrestees may underreport their use of illicit drugs; these low rates of self-reported concurrent use of illicit methadone, however, were supported by results of voluntary urine tests. Very small percentages of male and female booked arrestees tested positive for methadone in 1992: for males, 2 percent or less; for females, 4 percent or less. New York is again a striking exception; in 1992, 7 percent of males and 11 percent of females tested positive for methadone. At the same time, the larger percentage of arrestees testing positive for methadone in New York, some of whose methadone programs have traditionally had liberal take-home policies, does suggest the association of such policies with a higher incidence of diversion, although at the same time the large number of methadone patients in New York does increase the likelihood that an arrestee will test positive for methadone. While higher than self-reports of street methadone use, the urinalysis data cannot distinguish between prescribed methadone and street methadone. Although the DUF questionnaire does ask whether the subject is currently in treatment, the type of treatment is not determined. But at worst, urinalysis results from DUF indicate that recent use of methadone among arrestees is low relative to other drugs included in the DUF study.

National AIDS Demonstration Research (NADR) Data

Another data source for street use of methadone comes from the NIDA funded National AIDS Demonstration Research (NADR) program (1987–1992)

---

[10] Thanks are due to Talbert Cottey, National Institute of Justice, for help in analyzing the DUF data and to Jessie Hsieh, UCLA Drug Abuse Research Center, for conducting the analysis of the data.

(also discussed in chapter 3).[11] The following discussion summarizes the results for injection drug users with respect to questions asked about "nonprescription methadone" (see Table 4-3). In an attempt to reflect possible differences in policy at the program or state level, results are also reported by U.S. census region. Overall, 27.3 percent of injection drug users said that they had used nonprescription methadone at some time in their life, and 3.6 percent had injected it.[12] In the prior 6 months, 11.6 percent had used it, but only 2.0 percent used it regularly, twice a week or more. As can be seen from Table 4-3, use of street methadone was about twice as high in the Northeast as in other regions of the country.

The "ever used" figures in Table 4-3 are considerably higher than those shown for the DUF results in Table 4-2. The difference is largely accounted for by the differences in the sample characteristics:The NADR subjects included in the above analysis were all injection drug users; by contrast, the DUF subjects were arrestees. The NADR sample includes a much higher percentage of hard-core, long-term drug users, who are more likely to have had experience with street methadone than the diverse subjects interviewed in DUF. However, even in this high drug use population, about 2 percent used street methadone twice a week or more.

---

[11] Eligibility criteria for respondents were as follows: (1) 18 years or older for programs funded in 1987, and 13 years or older for programs funded in 1988; (2) injection of drugs in the past six months; and/or (3) sexual relations with an injection drug user within the past six months; and (4) not enrolled in treatment within the past 30 days. Using these criteria, respondents were classified as an injection drug user or as the sex partner of an injection drug user. (Since the former took precedence in client classification, none of the sex partners had injected drugs within the past six months). Participants were recruited mainly through community outreach in 5p sites. Most (80 percent) of the interviews were conducted in 1989 or 1990. Initial interviews were conducted with 43,443 injection drug users and with 9,791 sex partners. (The NADR public use data tape and documentation were provided by Richard Needle, Ph.D., M.P.H., Community Research Branch, National Institute on Drug Abuse. Thanks are due to Mel Widawski, Senior Statistician, UCLA Drug Abuse Research Center, for data analysis, and to Helen Cesare, Community Research Branch, National Institute on Drug Abuse, for reviewing the results of the analysis.)

[12] Of these, 95 percent reported having ever used nonprescription methadone by noninjection and 13 percent by injection (the wording of the questionnaire accounts for the overlap in responses).

TABLE 4-3 Percentage of Injection Drug Users Reporting Nonprescription Methadone Use in NADR Program Initial Interview, 1989–1990, by Region and in Total

U.S. Census Region	Ever Used			Used in Past 6 Months (Noninjection Only)			
	Non-injection	In-jection	Both	Any	<4 a Month	Once a Week	2+ a Week
Northeast	39.9	3.6	40.8	22.2	13.7	4.8	3.8
North Central	18.8	4.2	20.6	6.1	4.0	1.0	1.0
South	18.7	3.7	20.1	6.9	4.8	1.0	1.2
West	22.7	5.1	24.4	8.5	6.0	1.0	1.5
Puerto Rico	18.7	0.5	18.9	5.0	2.8	1.1	1.2
Total	26.0	3.6	27.3	11.6	7.5	2.1	2.0

NOTE: NADR = National AIDS Demonstration Research program. $N = 43,443$.

HOW IS METHADONE DIVERTED?

Potentially, methadone gets into the illicit market in various ways, including importation from other countries, clandestine domestic manufacture, thefts at various points in the manufacture and distribution system, excess physician dispensing, thefts by clinic staff, clinic patients' sales of their dosages, and theft of patients' take-home doses. The following discussion attempts to provide some indication of the importance of each of these.

Estimates of the amount of methadone that is diverted per year are not available. Since most of the methadone diverted comes from patients, largely in the form of take-home doses, and since DEA does not prosecute street-level dealers, the agency makes no effort to determine the quantities of methadone diverted (A.L. Carter, DEA, personal communication, April 15, 1994). Such estimates would be useful in assessing the degree of harm that diverted methadone might be causing.

Production and Distribution System

DEA security and record-keeping requirements for schedule II drugs keep leakage of methadone from the production, distribution, and storage points to a minimum. In 1977, 18,000 methadone dosage units were reported stolen from in-transit vehicles, programs, or other sources; this represents sources less than 0.06 percent of the 31,000,000 dosage units dispensed in treatment programs (based on a standard dosage unit of 40 mg) (U.S. Congress, 1978). The rarity of thefts of substantial amounts of methadone has led federal drug enforcement officials to conclude that the traditional sources of illicit drugs—smuggling from other countries, domestic illicit manufacture, and distribution by organized crime—play little or no role in the marketing of street methadone.

Sale by Patients: Who Sells and Why?

Since 1974, when the Narcotic Addict Treatment Act of 1974 effectively ended indiscriminate script writing by physicians, the sale of methadone by program patients has been regarded as the main avenue by which methadone reaches the street market. To collect ethnographic data on street sale and use of methadone, in 1981–1982, Spunt et al. (1986) conducted a study of methadone diversion through interviews with 247 subjects drawn from three groups located in three northeastern states:patients in methadone treatment programs, current narcotic users not in treatment, and patients recently withdrawn from methadone. Additional data came from observations by research staff and informal interviews conducted at the programs and in the surrounding areas. The study provided information on two main questions:Who sells diverted methadone? Who buys diverted methadone?

Spunt and his colleagues found that program staff accounted for a very small amount of the diverted methadone, partly because DEA security and record-keeping requirements made such diversion very difficult. Procedures for delivering methadone from wholesalers to individual programs also made it unlikely that in-transit methadone was diverted to the street market in any significant quantity.

Patients, according to Spunt, were found to be the main source of diverted methadone, through sales of either take-home medication or "spitbacks" (medication held in the mouth rather than swallowed and spit into a container after leaving the clinic). At the time the study was conducted, a take-home bottle of 50 mg cost between $15 and $25 on the street, with the price varying with the amount of methadone in the area, the day of the week, and program policy.[13] The less desirable "spitbacks" cost less than take-home doses. Spitting back was more likely to occur at programs where take-home privileges were kept to a minimum, and where there were no other methadone programs nearby.

While one-third of patients interviewed had sold their medication at least once, only 10 percent (23) did so regularly. The two most common reasons given by these regular diverters were to make money (often to buy other drugs) and to provide methadone to a spouse or a friend who needed it.

Spunt and his colleagues concluded that regular diversion of methadone can be attributed to three main interrelated factors: (1) continued drug use (of heroin or other drugs) by patients, (2) the need to supplement income, and (3) the desire to share with or sell the diverted methadone to an addicted friend or spouse.[14] Although there are a number of motives or reasons for selling or sharing methadone, and these may differ at different times for the same individual, the small number of people in this study who regularly sold methadone makes it difficult to determine the relative importance of the various motives among methadone diverters generally.

WHO USES DIVERTED METHADONE AND WHY?

The study by Spunt and his colleagues (1986) also collected data on the characteristics of buyers of diverted methadone and why they used it. Most buyers of street methadone were heroin addicts who were either unwilling or unable to enter treatment. Over half of the sample of heroin users not currently in treatment reported that they used illicit methadone in the week before the interview, 60 percent of these to eliminate withdrawal symptoms, and the remainder to get "high."

The researchers identified a number of reasons for using street methadone:

• To substitute for heroin when heroin supplies are low, when prices are high, or when it is inconvenient or difficult to contact a dealer;
• To avoid formal treatment when wishing to withdraw from heroin or to create an unsupervised program;

---

[13] As an example of the effect of program policy, in one city illicit supplies of methadone increased when a program dismissed many of its maintenance patients for nonpayment of fees. Presumably, this group increased demand for illegal methadone.

[14] To the reasons identified by the Spunt study, may be added another: In any area where patients must pay for treatment, they may sell methadone to help pay for treatment (Rosenbaum, Murphy, & Beck, 1987).

- To experience the euphoric effects of methadone; [15]
- To supplement the methadone prescribed by the program, either to eliminate withdrawal symptoms resulting from an inadequate dose of methadone or to experience euphoria from "double dosing."

There is some reason to believe that those who supplement their prescribed doses of methadone do so because the low doses provided by some programs as a matter of policy do not "hold" them for 24 hours. Thus, such programs may encourage a street market for methadone among their patients. While the current movement toward more adequate dosing practices may help to reduce this factor in diversion, it may also enable patients who find the low doses sufficient to divert part of their prescribed doses.

From the results of this study, as well as earlier studies, it appears that street methadone is more often used by heroin addicts and methadone-maintained patients as a form of self-medication than to produce euphoria (to get high).

CONSEQUENCES OF METHADONE DIVERSION

The consequences of methadone diversion fall into two broad areas: public safety and public health.

Public Safety Issues

The sale or distribution of methadone outside of the closed system of registered manufacturers, wholesalers, hospitals, pharmacies, and programs is illegal. The public has a right to expect that federal agencies will enforce the provisions of the Controlled Substances Act and its implementing regulations. There is no information on the degree to which methadone is implicated in drug-related crime or how much police effort is devoted to the prevention of its diversion. The lack of such information suggests that diverted methadone plays a small part in the overall drug-crime problem and receives a low priority in law enforcement efforts.

---

[15] For 13 percent of the narcotic addicts in the Spunt study not in treatment (n = 142), methadone was the main drug taken for its euphoric effect.

Public Health Issues

Is Diverted Methadone Dangerous?

To what extent, and under what circumstances, does methadone cause or contribute to death and morbidity? In assessing the meaning of "methadone-related death," as noted above, it is important to determine whether methadone detected in the decedent was taken during treatment or obtained on the street. It is also important to know the cause of death. Is death due to an overdose of methadone or to some other cause having little or nothing to do with methadone? And do drug overdose deaths in which methadone is present generally involve simultaneous toxic levels of other drugs? If drugs other than methadone are detected in a overdose case, how is the contribution, if any, of methadone determined? We noted earlier that there is no strong evidence that methadone plays an important role in drug-related deaths or emergency hospital care. Because methadone is taken orally in the vast majority of cases (96 percent), it does not expose users to the hazards consequent on injection with nonsterile needles, which play such an important role in heroin's contribution to disease and death. However, diverted methadone would be expected to have the same adverse side effects as does clinic-dispensed methadone (see chapter 2).

DEA argues that the income from street methadone is used to purchase other illicit drugs. If these other drugs are then injected, the risk to the public health is increased. Data to support this argument are not available. Indeed, in the absence of reliable data, it is impossible to arrive at a clear assessment of any potential public effects of diverted methadone. At the very least, the extent and consequences of methadone diversion need to be considered carefully in any assessment of the public health benefits and risks of diversion.

Is Diverted Methadone a Major Drug of Abuse?

The data presented above from DAWN, DUF, and other sources indicate that while methadone has some potential for abuse when diverted from normal channels, the extent of the abuse associated with diverted methadone is small relative to heroin and cocaine. While methadone has a high addiction liability, instances of primary methadone addiction are few. Thus, while some street methadone is abused, it constitutes a relatively small part of the drug abuse problem generally.

SUMMARY

DEA and FDA regulations and their implementation reduced the metha-done diversion that existed in the early 1970s. In addition, clinical practices and procedures have contributed to keeping methadone diversion at a low level. Although practices vary from clinic to clinic, the following are in common use:(1) Upon entry of patients to treatment, counselors discuss, among other things, dosing procedures, take-home polices, and procedures for dealing with diverting methadone; (2) regular clinic patients present an identification card that indicates program enrollment; (3) the methadone dose is diluted with water and patients are required to drink all of it, which makes it difficult to retain in the mouth; (4) patients take their methadone dose under observation and the nurse asks the patient to speak afterwards, which discourages "spitbacks"; (5) cups or other containers are not allowed in the dosing area; (6) waiting and dispensing areas are separated, which helps the monitoring of medication ingestion; (7) patients receiving take-home doses are required to return with empty bottles, and clinics may make random calls to ask that all issued bottles (empty and filled) be brought in for inspection; (8) urine samples are tested for the presence of the methadone metabolite, which discourages diversion by those with take-home doses; and (9) any patient observed, or otherwise known to be, selling methadone is subject to clinic disciplinary action, including a fair hearing, but which may involve discharge from the program.

However, as long as patients are allowed to take weekend doses home, and as long as programs reward long-term compliance with program rules with greater take-home privileges, there is a potential for patient-initiated diversion. Even without "take-homes," some patients would continue to pretend to swallow a dose in the clinic but manage to save it and expel it for sale after they leave the premises. Other potential sources of diverted methadone are thefts, hijackings, and robberies at the various distribution points. The evidence reviewed above, however, indicates that the amount of methadone diverted to the street, through whatever means, is relatively small.

What happens to diverted methadone? Methadone has rarely been the preferred drug of abuse by users of illegal drugs. Its action is too slow, and the level of euphoria it provides, particularly when taken orally, is too mild for most drug users to select it over other opiates. Rather, it has mainly served as a way to avoid or end withdrawal symptoms, as a form of self-treatment for heroin addiction, or as a substitute for heroin or other opiates when they are in short supply.

How much medical harm does diverted methadone do? Although methadone has the potential to cause death in individuals who lack tolerance to it or opiates in general, its use primarily by individuals who are dependent on, and tolerant to, opiates results in minimal medical harm. Although the risk of medical harm of street methadone is greatest for nontolerant persons, the number of cases in which methadone has been documented as the sole direct cause of death is very small.

Chapter one reviewed the evidence on the effectiveness of methadone maintenance treatment. Briefly, research conducted over the past 30 years has indicated positive outcomes from methadone maintenance, including reductions in illicit opiate use, in criminal activity, and in risk of disease, death, and HIV transmission, and increases in socially productive activities. These beneficial outcomes have been obtained despite the highly restrictive regulatory environment, primarily to control methadone diversion.

In the main, the committee concludes, on the basis of the available data and the experience of its clinician and researcher members, that should FDA regulations be changed in the ways recommended in chapter 7, the potential increase in methadone diversion would be small because of its intrinsic lack of attractiveness compared with other drugs of abuse. This belief rests on limited data and thus the committee recommends careful monitoring of effects of the suggested changes with a plan to act quickly to reinstate restrictions if diversion becomes a major health problem. Further, the committee concludes that the risks to the public safety and the public health of diverted methadone do not outweigh the benefits of making methadone treatment more readily available.

Finally, the approval, in 1993, of LAAM for the treatment of opiate addiction by the FDA is related to the issue of diversion. Owing to its long duration of action, patients only need to take LAAM three times a week rather than every day. In addition, LAAM's slow onset of action virtually eliminates the possibility of getting "high," thus greatly reducing its demand on the street as a drug of abuse. FDA regulations for LAAM, which now form a section of the original methadone regulations (as described in chapter 5), do not allow for any take-homes doses. As the use of LAAM becomes more common in the treatment of opiate addiction, there may be a reduction in the number of patients receiving methadone (assuming no significant increase in funding for opiate agonist pharmacotherapy), with a corresponding decrease in methadone diversion. At the same time, concern for methadone diversion may have influenced FDA's decision to prohibit LAAM take-homes, even though LAAM has advantages as a take-home medication in terms of its lower diversion risk and abuse potential.

APPENDIX

Harris County, Texas

A Centers for Disease Control (CDC) investigation was prompted by events in Harris County, Texas. In 1991, a reported rise in the number of methadone-related deaths in Harris County led to increased scrutiny by authorities over local methadone treatment programs. Most methadone treatment programs in Houston and the surrounding areas are private, and for-profit, having been developed to fill the void left when local government abandoned the service delivery of methadone treatment. Federal regulators began investigating the claim that methadone-related deaths were occurring from illicit methadone originating from poorly monitored methadone treatment programs. Liberal methadone take-home policies were blamed for creating a situation where addicts could sell their surplus methadone on the black market. These problems prompted a six-month joint investigation by DEA, FDA, and the Texas Department of Health.

In March 1992, acting on the basis of an undercover purchase of illicit methadone, DEA ordered a privately owned, for-profit methadone clinic in Houston to show cause why its license to dispense methadone should not be suspended. The clinic was closed and this closure was soon followed by similar orders to close two more clinics—all three owned by the same person. DEA orders to close these three clinics were described in a series of articles by the *Houston Chronicle* (e.g., "Methadone Clinic Shut in Raid Here," March 19, 1992, and "2d Methadone Facility Shuts Down," April 10, 1992), which were distributed over the national wire services and publicized widely. The articles also reported, quite inaccurately, that methadone was killing nearly twice as many people in the Houston area as was heroin, which was attributed to poorly run methadone clinics.

In November 1992, prompted by reports of an increase in the number of methadone-related deaths in Harris County in 1991, the Texas Department of Health and the Interagency Methadone Policy Review Board, a committee composed of representatives from all federal agencies involved in oversight of methadone treatment, invited the CDC to investigate the deaths in Harris County. The CDC investigation was the most careful and comprehensive of recent investigations into methadone-related deaths.

The incidents in Texas (but not including the CDC investigation, which was then in progress) received nationwide television attention on February 21, 1993, when CBS News, on "60 Minutes," broadcast a segment entitled "Just Say Yes." In this segment, "60 Minutes" focused on DEA-enforced closures of the three Houston methadone maintenance clinics and stressed the public and political opposition to methadone maintenance treatment. The "60 Minute" report focused on the Houston controversy, arguing that when methadone treatment of Heroin addicts became a for-profit, money-making business, the emphasis shifted from detoxification to maintenance.

REFERENCES

Barrett, DH, Luk, AJ, Parrish, G, and Jones, TS. 1993. *Medical examiner cases in which methadone was detected, Harris County, Texas, 1987–1992.* Unpublished report. Atlanta, Centers for Disease Control and Prevention.

Chambers, CD, and Bergen, JJ. 1973. Self-administered methadone supplementation. In: C. D. Chambers and L. Brill (eds.), *Methadone: Experiences and Issues.* New York: Behavioral Publications. Pp. 131–142.

Chambers, CD, and Inciardi, JA. 1972. An empirical assessment of the availability of illicit methadone. In: *Proceedings,* Fourth National Conference on Methadone Treatment, San Francisco, January 8–10. Pp. 149–151.

Courtwright, DT. 1992. A century of American narcotic policy. In: D. R. Gerstein and H. J. Harwood (eds.), *Treating Drug Problems.* Vol. 2. Washington, D.C.: National Academy Press. Pp. 1–62).

Dole, VP, and Nyswander, M. 1965. A medical treatment for diacetylmorphine (heroin) addiction. *Journal of the American Medical Association* 193:80–84

General Accounting Office. 1976. *More Effective Action Needed to Control Abuse and Diversion in Methadone Treatment Programs: Food and Drug Administration, Department of Health, Education and Welfare, Drug Enforcement Administration, Department of Justice.* GGD-76-51. Washington, D.C.: Government Printing Office.

General Accounting Office. 1990. *Methadone Maintenance: Some Treatment Programs Are Not Effective.* HRD-90-104. Washington, D.C.: U.S. Government Printing Office.

Gottschalk, LA, McGuire, FL, Dinovo, EC, Birch, H, and Heiser, JF. 1977. *Guide to the Investigation and Reporting of Drug-Abuse Deaths.* DHEW Publication No. (ADM) 77-386. Rockville, Md.: National Institute on Drug Abuse.

Gottschalk, LA, McGuire, FL, Heiser, JF, Dinovo, EC, and Birch, H. 1979. *Drug Abuse Deaths in Nine Cities: A Survey Report.* NIDA Research Monograph 29, Rockville, Md.

Gottschalk, LA, and Cravey, RH. 1980. *Toxicological and Pathological Studies on Psychoactive Drug-Involved Deaths.* Davis, Calif.: Biomedical Publications.

Inciardi, JA. 1977. *Methadone Diversion: Experiences and Issues.* Rockville, Md.: National Institute on Drug Abuse.

Karch, S. 1993. *The Pathology of Drug Abuse.* Boca Raton, Fla.: CRC Press.

Martin, JM, Quinn, TM, and Bonacum, WT. 1975. *Methadone diversion II: A second study in five cities.* Unpublished manuscript. Bronx, N.Y.: Fordham University, Institute for Social Research.

Martin, JM, Quinn, TM, and McCahey, JP. 1973. *Methadone Diversion: A Study in Five Cities.* Rockville: National Institute on Drug Abuse.

Musto, DF. 1987. *The American Disease: Origins of Narcotic Control.* (Expanded edition.) New York: Oxford University Press.

National Institute on Drug Abuse. 1977. *Drug Watch: July 1977.* DHEW Publication No. (ADM) 77-503. Rockville, Md.: NIDA.

National Institute on Drug Abuse. 1989. NIDA's methadone diversion field investiga tion, October 3–4, 1989. Unpublished report (October 6).

Project DAWN III. 1976. Washington, D.C.: Drug Enforcement Administration and National Institute of Drug Abuse.

Rosenbaum, M, Murphy, S, and Beck, J. 1987. Money for methadone: Preliminary findings from a study of Alameda County's new maintenance policy. *Journal of Psychoactive Drugs* 19(1):13–19.

Sapira, JD, Ball, JC, and Cottrell, ES. 1973. Methadone as a primary drug of addiction. In: C. D. Chambers and L. Brill (eds.), *Methadone: Experiences and Issues.* New York: Behavioral Publications. Pp. 87–93.

Spunt, B, Hunt, D, Lipton, DS, and Goldsmith, DS. 1986. Methadone diversion: A new look. *Journal of Drug Issues* 18(4):569–583.

Stephens, RC, and Weppner, RS. 1973a. Legal and illegal use of methadone: One year later. *American Journal of Psychiatry* 130(12):1391–1394.

Stephens, RC, and Weppner, RS. 1973b. Patterns of "cheating" among methadone maintenance patients. *Drug Forum,* 2(4):357–366.

U.S. House of Representative. 1973. Committee on Interstate and Foreign Commerce. Subcommittee on Public Health and Environment (1973). *Regulation of Methadone and Other Narcotic Drugs in Treatment Programs.* Hearings, June 18 and 27, 1973. 93rd Cong., 1st sess. (Serial No. 93-29)

U.S. Senate. 1973c. Committee on the Judiciary. Subcommittee to Investigate Juvenile Delinquency. *Methadone Use and Abuse: 1972–1973.* Hearings, November 14 and 16, 1972; February 8, 13, and 14, and April 5, 1973. 92nd Cong., 2nd sess., and 93rd Cong., 1st sess.

U.S. Senate. 1973b. Committee on the Judiciary. *Methadone Diversion Control Act of 1973.* 93rd Cong., 1st sess. June 4, 1973. (Report 93-192)

U.S. House of Representatives. 1978. Select Committee on Narcotics Abuse and Control. *Methadone Diversion:A Report.* 95th Cong., 2nd sess. (SCNAC-95-2-17)

U.S. House of Representatives. 1989. Select Committee on Narcotics Abuse and Control. *Efficacy of Drug Abuse Treatment Programs.* Hearings, July 25, August 2, 1989. 101st Cong., 1st sess.

U.S. House of Representatives. 1990. Select Committee on Narcotics Abuse and Control. 1990. *Hearing on Methadone Treatment and Drug Addiction.* March 23, 1990. 101st Cong., 2nd sess. (SCNAC-101-2-7)

Walter, PV, Sheridan, BK, and Chambers, CD. 1973. Methadone diversion: A study in illicit availability. In C. D. Chambers and L. Brill (eds.), *Methadone: Experiences and Issues.* New York: Behavioral Publications. Pp. 171–176.

Weppner, RS, and Stephens, RC. 1973. The illicit use and diversion of methadone on the street as related by hospitalized addicts. *Journal of Drug Issues* 3:42–47.

Weppner, RS, Stephens, RC, and Conrad, HT. 1972. Methadone: Some aspects of its legal and illegal use. *American Journal of Psychiatry* 129:111–115.

Wright, C. 1992. *Medical Officer Briefing Package: The Houston Methadone Outbreak.* Rockville, Md.: Food and Drug Administration.

5

Federal Regulation of Methadone Treatment

The roots of the concurrent regulation of certain drugs under two statutory schemes go back to the beginning of this century. In 1906, Congress enacted the Pure Food and Drug Act, establishing one regime of regulation to assure (among other things) that drugs were not adulterated or misbranded. These regulations were amended several times, recodified in 1938, and expanded on again from the 1940s through the 1990s. Their implementation and enforcement is today assigned to the Food and Drug Administration (FDA) in the Department of Health and Human Services (DHHS).

In 1914, Congress adopted the Harrison Narcotic Act to stop abuse of addictive drugs. The Harrison Narcotic Act was amended in 1937 to include marijuana. In 1965, amphetamines, barbiturates, and hallucinogens came under regulation, but under the Federal Food, Drug, and Cosmetic Act. In 1970, these various statutes were consolidated and recodified as the Controlled Substances Act (CSA), which has been amended several times since then. Its implementation and enforcement is today assigned to the Drug Enforcement Administration (DEA) in the Department of Justice.

In short, two distinct regulatory schemes—one based on truth-in-labeling to protect consumers using drugs for medical purposes, the other based on limiting access altogether to protect the public from drugs of abuse—have grown up in parallel for 80 years. About 75 years ago, and again 25 years ago, the traditions underpinning each scheme came together and conflicted. The issue each time was whether opiate addicts should be given an opiate to "maintain" their addictions.[1]

---

[1]"Maintain" here simply means provide methadone for a period longer than the minimum required to detoxify the addict from heroin or opiate use and long enough to wean him or her off methadone itself without greatly debilitating physical symptoms.

The first clash occurred after World War I, when so-called "morphine clinics" existed and physicians prescribed or dispensed morphine to addicts. Some addicts were veterans of the American Civil War, the Spanish-American War, and WWI, who had become addicted during treatment for war wounds, but most of them came from the growing population of nonmedical addicts (Courtwright, 1982). The Narcotics Division of the Prohibition Unit of the Department of the Treasury, which was then responsible for enforcing the Harrison Narcotic Act, concluded that this activity was not the legitimate practice of medicine but simple drug trafficking. The Treasury Department swiftly closed the clinics and made it personally and professionally risky for physicians to "maintain" a narcotic addict for any reason. In did so, however, only after the American Medical Association had adopted a resolution, in 1920, opposing "ambulatory clinics" (Musto, 1987, p. 148)

This story, as summarized above, became part of the "lore" that affected medical practice and research for almost 50 years and had a profound influence on government officials when the issue of narcotic maintenance again emerged in relation to methadone. In 1972, the public health establishment, including the Secretary of Health, Education, and Welfare, the Food and Drug Administration, the National Institute of Mental Health, and the Special Action Office for Drug Abuse Prevention, was unprepared to allow the Bureau of Narcotics and Dangerous Drugs, DEA's predecessor agency, to unilaterally define the parameters of medical practice for the use of methadone in the treatment of heroin addiction. *As a consequence*, a new set of rules—the third, on top of the FDA and DEA schemes—was added, one that inserted FDA deeply into the practice of medicine, notwithstanding its protestations to the contrary. Congress ratified this joint responsibility of law enforcement and public health officials for methadone through this third set of rules in 1974 with the passage of the Narcotic Addict Treatment Act (NATA). To examine in detail the evolution of this third set of rules—commonly referred to as the FDA or DHHS methadone regulations—we turn, first, to the period of the mid-1960s.

THE 1960s

Increased use of heroin in the post World War II period first became apparent in the early to mid 1950s. By the end of that decade, New York City had established a special program for young people. The U.S. Public Health Service hospital at Lexington, Kentucky, admitted a number of unemancipated minors from major eastern U.S. metropolitan areas. And during the Eisenhower Administration, a minimum mandatory narcotics law was enacted in 1956, effective July 1957.

In the 1960s, the use of amphetamines and marijuana, in addition to heroin, increased rapidly, especially among younger persons. From the mid-1960s onward, however, concern about heroin use among inner city residents began to displace earlier concern about psychopharmacological drugs of pleasure. The unfolding policy response to these events included a 1962 White House conference on drug abuse, the President's Advisory Committee on Narcotic and Drug Abuse (the Prettyman Committee) of 1963, the Drug Abuse Control Amendments of 1965, the President's Commission on Law Enforcement and Administration of Justice (the Katzenbach Commission) of 1966–1967, and the Narcotic Addiction Rehabilitation Act of 1966.

The 1965 Drug Abuse Control Amendments brought under strict federal control all nonnarcotic drugs capable of producing serious psychotoxic effects when abused. This act also created the Bureau of Drug Abuse Control within the Department of Health, Education, and Welfare (DHEW) and shifted the basis for federal law enforcement of illegal drugs from tax principles (administered by the Department of Treasury) to the regulation of commerce (administered by the DHEW).

The 1966 Narcotic Addiction Rehabilitation Act (NARA) authorized the civil commitment of narcotic addicts, and federal assistance to state and local governments to develop a local system of drug treatment programs. With respect to the latter, the National Institute of Mental Health (NIMH) initially proposed the gradual implementation of the state assistance effort, mainly through a common mental health mechanism—inpatient treatment programs. However, because of a perceived pressing need, the courts began to commit addicts to these programs even before they were officially opened or staffed. Overwhelmed, most programs were forced to provide less costly services on an outpatient basis, which subsequently became the primary setting for addiction treatment. (Courtwright, 1992; Bestamen, 1992) The NARA legislation imposed the following contract requirements on treatment centers: (1) thrice-a-week counseling sessions; (2) weekly urine tests; (3) restorative dental services; (4) psychological consultations and vocational training; and (5) the treatment modalities of drug-free outpatient, therapeutic community, and methadone maintenance (interview of Karst Besteman by Richard A. Rettig, December 20, 1993; hereafter Besteman interview[2]).

These policy developments were accompanied by changes in the federal agencies responsible for narcotics. Reorganization Plan No. 1 of 1968 transferred the primary functions of the Federal Bureau of Narcotics (FBN) from the Treasury Department to the Department of Justice; it also transferred the DHEW Bureau of Drug Abuse Control functions to the Department of

---

[2]Karst Besteman was deputy director of the NIMH Division of Narcotic Addiction and Drug Abuse in the late 1960s and early 1970s.

Justice. Within the Justice Department, the Bureau of Narcotics and Dangerous Drugs (BNDD) was created, which became the Drug Enforcement Administration in 1973. DHEW responsibilities for narcotic addiction treatment were lodged in the NIMH. The NIMH nucleus eventually became the basis for the National Institute on Drug Abuse.

THE NIXON ADMINISTRATION

Under the first Nixon administration (1969–1972), federal drug abuse policy developed in a significant way. These developments included a 1969 "war on drugs" presidential message, resulting legislation in 1970, and a Special Action Office created by executive order in 1971 and authorized in statute in 1972.

The perception that the heroin problem in the United States was an epidemic was reinforced at the end of the 1960s and during the early 1970s by the widespread exposure of GIs in Vietnam to the drug. A fear arose that many GIs, sent to Vietnam often against their will and over the protests of many of their countrymen, would return not as conquering heroes but as heroin addicts.

This prospect, plus the public concern with crime and the association of crime and illegal drug use, led President Nixon, in 1969, to send a message to Congress on drug abuse. Although this was the first time that a U.S. president invoked the "war on drugs" image, it was in retrospect the most balanced approach to the problem of drug abuse that had been advanced. Although Nixon's blueprint gave highest priority to supply reduction, it also placed strong emphasis on demand reduction, more so than did any subsequent administration.

1970 Legislation

The 1969 message resulted in the submission of legislation to the Congress and the passage, the following year, of the Comprehensive Drug Abuse Prevention and Control Act of 1970 (Public Law 91-513, October 27, 1970). The act dealt with research, treatment, and prevention of drug abuse and drug dependence, and with drug abuse law enforcement authority.

One major purpose of the 1970 legislation was to reverse some of the strictures of the Harrison Act of 1914. The 1970 act sought "to clarify for the medical profession . . . the extent to which they may safely go in treating narcotic addicts as patients. There are relatively few practicing physicians in the U.S. today who treat narcotic addicts because of the uncertainty as to the extent to which they may prescribe narcotic drugs for addict patients." (U.S.

House of Representatives, 1970). In this regard, Congress was redressing the interpretation of the Harrison Act that followed upon the closing of the morphine clinics some fifty years earlier.

To achieve this clarification, Title I, in Section IV, charged the Secretary of Health, Education, and Welfare, to "determine the appropriate methods of professional practice in the medical treatment of the narcotic addiction of various classes of narcotic addicts." This provision constitutes the initial statutory basis for treatment standards. More important, it clearly stated that the health establishment, *not* the law enforcement community, would determine the scope of the practice of medicine in this area.

The law enforcement sections consolidated all prior federal statutes into the Controlled Substances Act and the Controlled Substances Export and Import Act (Titles II and III, respectively, of the Comprehensive Drug Abuse Prevention and Control Act of 1970). Under this legislation, substances were classified under five schedules "according to their abuse potential, and psychological and physical effects." Methadone was placed in Schedule II, along with such opiate drugs as morphine, codeine, and hydrocodone.

Special Action Office for Drug Abuse Presentation

One of the most important steps taken by President Nixon was to establish in June 1971 the Special Action Office for Drug Abuse Prevention (SAODAP) in the Executive Office of the President (By Executive Order 11,599, June 17, 1971). In mid-1971, Nixon appointed Dr. Jerome Jaffe as SAODAP director. Within a year, the Drug Abuse Prevention Office and Treatment Act of 1972 (Public Law 92-255, March 21, 1972) gave statutory authority to SAODAP, but limiting setting, on June 30, 1975, as the limit on its existence.

The purpose of the 1972 act was to bring the resources of the federal government to bear on drug abuse with the immediate objective of significantly reducing its incidence and developing a comprehensive, coordinated long-term federal strategy to combat drug abuse. The SAODAP direction thus became the "czar" for devising and executing strategies for reducing the demand for drugs. Title II, for example, authorized the director to: make grants and contracts; provide overall planning and policy for all federal drug abuse prevention functions; review current regulations, guidelines, criteria, requirements, and procedures of agencies for consistency with newly established policy; review related federal legislation to assure that all administering agencies viewed drug abuse as a health problem; and coordinate all federal departments and agencies in the fight against drug abuse.

Title III required the development of a national strategy directed by the President. Title IV amended the Community Mental Health Centers Act to include drug abuse treatment and rehabilitation among the array of services offered, to deny approval of any state plan that failed to provide for drug abuse and drug dependence treatment and prevention, and to bar denial of admission to or treatment to drug abusers in hospitals receiving federal funds solely because of their drug abuse or drug dependence.

Finally, Title V authorized the creation of the National Institute on Drug Abuse, within the NIMH, effective December 31, 1974, to develop and conduct comprehensive health, education, training, research, and planning programs for the prevention and treatment of drug abuse and for the rehabilitation of drug abusers. (NIDA was actually created in 1973, earlier than authorized, when NIMH, which had been moved out of the NIH in 1967, was reorganized as the Alcohol, Drug Abuse, and Mental Health Administration. The constituent agencies of the new ADAMHA became NIMH, NIDA, and the National Institute of Alcohol Abuse and Alcoholism.)

Although the Special Action Office did not exist when FDA issued regulations for methadone Investigational New Drugs (INDs) in 1971, it was significantly involved in the development of 1972 methadone regulations. Dr. Jaffe and his staff actively participated in the drafting of these regulations, in concert with FDA and BNDD staff, as well as in the writing of the 1974 Narcotic Addict Treatment Act. Since SAODAP also controlled federal funding of treatment programs, its role was very important in encouraging and nurturing the establishment and development of methadone treatment programs.

DEFINING THE REGULATORY REGIME: 1970–1974

The methadone regulatory regime—the third set of rules governing methadone treatment was defined in the period 1970 through 1974 by the Comprehensive Drug Abuse Prevention and Control Act of 1970, the FDA methadone regulations for Investigational New Drugs of 1971, the FDA methadone regulations of 1972, and the Narcotic Addict Treatment Act of 1974. We first deal briefly with the clinical antecedents to the FDA regulations, then consider their evolution.

Research, Treatment, and Regulation

Methadone was approved by FDA for use as an analgesic and antitussive (for prevention and suppression of coughing) on August 13, 1947, when a New

Drug Application (NDA 6134) was granted for Dolophine to Eli Lilly & Co.[3]
Methadone was first studied in this country in 1946 at the U.S. Public Health
Service Hospital in Lexington, Kentucky.[4] It was found to be similar to
morphine in its effects but possibly longer acting. Clinical research showed
that opiate withdrawal syndrome could be treated effectively by substituting
methadone for morphine and slowly reducing the dose over a 7–10 day period.
Its primary use in addiction treatment was to withdraw addicts from heroin,
well before methadone maintenance treatment was developed.

In 1962, Vincent Dole and Marie Nyswander at Rockefeller University
began planning clinical studies to use methadone with carefully selected
narcotic addicts in New York City. Their research, which started in late 1963,
and was first reported in Dole (1965), demonstrated that methadone could be
used to treat intractable heroin addicts by maintenance, not detoxification.

Beginning in the mid-1960s, the findings of Dole, Nyswander, and Mary
Jeanne Kreek were reported in a number of papers (Dole, et al., 1966). As a
result, many interested researchers and clinicians visited Rockefeller to learn
about their treatment protocols. Annual conferences, held from 1968 through
1971, and sponsored by the National Association for the Prevention of
Addiction to Narcotics, resulted in the rapid dissemination of this research and
the creation of a close professional network to promote the use of methadone
in treating heroin addiction (Besteman interview).

The course of the transition from clinical research to greater use of
methadone for treatment was unusual, however. In 1947, when FDA approved
Lilly's NDA for methadone, it required only the demonstration of safety under
the 1938 Federal Food, Drug, and Cosmetic Act (FFDCA). The 1962
amendments to the FFDCA added the requirement that FDA also evaluate the
effectiveness of new drugs before their introduction to the market. Although
the use of methadone for treating narcotic addiction was a new "indication for
use" that fell under the effectiveness requirement of the 1962 amendments,
FDA did not become deeply involved in its evaluation until the late 1960s and
early 1970s.

The normal route for seeking approval of a new drug or a "new indication" is for the sponsor of the drug (usually its manufacturer) to obtain an
Investigational New Drug (IND) authorization. Under an IND, evidence of
safety and effectiveness based on well-controlled clinical studies is developed
in support of an NDA (or a Supplemental NDA in the case of a new indication

---

[3]"Dolophine" was derived from "dolor" for pain. The street name for dolophine,
which is a wafer form of methadone, is "dolly." A persistent but false belief is that the
name derives from Adolf Hitler.

[4]It is worth noting that the Public Health Service was engaged in addiction research
well before the adoption in 1966 of the Narcotic Addict Rehabilitation Act.

for a previously approved drug). This course was not initially pursued in the case of methadone, perhaps because FDA was in the early stages of implementing the 1962 act and also because there was no pharmaceutical sponsor.

Dole's planning in the mid-1960s included an assessment of the legal authority of Rockefeller University to conduct such research. Although Dole and Nyswander's studies provided the clinical demonstration of effectiveness, they were not done under an IND, as FDA rules did not require one.[5] Dole viewed the Treasury's Bureau of Narcotics (FBN) as the primary federal agency that might have regulatory authority over his proposed research, and the key question was whether research using methadone to maintain heroin addicts as part of a treatment program in New York City was within the domain of the professional practice of medicine or was another form of trafficking, as FBN had claimed with respect to the morphine clinics some 40 years earlier (Dole, 1989).

After extensive consultation with university lawyers and officials, Dole concluded that prior Supreme Court decisions did not bar the use of methadone in "in the course of professional treatment." The FBN view, however, was that maintenance of narcotic addiction with any narcotic drug fell outside the normal course of professional treatment. Dole recalls a visit by an FBN agent who informed him that he was breaking the law and that he would be put in jail. Dole challenged his visitor to have the agency sue him, a distinguished member of the faculty of Rockefeller University. Nonplussed, the agent left, only to return a short time later with the message that the research could be conducted, but only under direction of the Bureau. Dole, secure in his knowledge of the limits of FBN authority, rejected this concession as well (telephone interview with Dr. Vincent Dole, December 1993). For roughly a five-year period, from 1965 through 1970, Dole's research went forward, harassed by the FBN, as Dole recalls, but without regulatory encumbrances.

---

[5]Before August 1962, no one had to file an IND with FDA; one simply had to comply with certain labeling and record-keeping requirements. The 1962 amendments expanded the IND provisions of the FFDCA and, even before the act was signed, FDA issued new regulations that required IND filings with FDA. Even under the new regulations, FDA did not attempt to require an IND for an individual physician who used a drug for research (or for a medical use other than FDA-approved), *if* the drug was in compliance with the law before the physician got it. Thus, methadone manufactured by Lilly and shipped to Rockefeller University's pharmacy and labeled in accord with the Lilly NDA was "lawful."

Methadone IND Regulations

During the mid to late 1960s, the period when Dole's results were beginning to attract the interest of researchers and clinicians, the FDA for its part showed little interest in the use of methadone. It simultaneously resisted the submission of an NDA for methadone on the grounds that there were no supporting scientific data developed under INDs, and did little to encourage IND submissions, with some FDA officials expressing skepticism that Dole was realizing the results being claimed (Besteman interview).

In a direct challenge to this situation, however, Dr. Sidney Cohen, director of the NIMH's Division of Narcotic Addiction and Drug Abuse (DNADA) in 1968–1969, applied for an IND for methadone clinical research (Besteman interview). A distinguished clinician and researcher who had come to government service from University of California, Los Angeles, Cohen was granted an IND. Out of concern that investigators participating under the Cohen IND be reputable and responsible, Cohen, and Dr. Richard Phillipson, his co-investigator, restricted them to NIMH grantees. The participants, who may have numbered as many as 15 to 20, reflected diverse philosophies of treatment; for example, Dr. William Wieland in Philadelphia advocated high doses of methadone, while Dr. Ray Knowles in St. Louis was more conservative. NIMH grantees were funded mainly by direct grants from DNADA, with most of the grants going directly to community mental health centers. Later, in the mid-1970s, funds were channeled through NIDA-funded state drug treatment programs.

Given Dole's results, and following the Cohen IND, other physicians sought and received INDs, with relatively little difficulty; FDA has indicated that more than 300 INDs were issued. In the eyes of the FDA, the situation was getting out of control. Consequently, in 1970, as controlled substances legislation was moving through Congress, the FDA sought to strengthen its control over the methadone treatment being conducted under INDs.

Although the IND-based research generated data on the use of methadone for treatment, these data were insufficient to justify the drug's approval as safe and effective and FDA concluded that further research was needed. It issued a proposed rule dealing with IND protocols for methadone treatment on June 11, 1970 (35 FR 9014). On April 2, 1971, a final rule of 2 1/2 pages specified the conditions of investigational use; the rule also responded to a BNDD regulation on IND requirements for controlled substances (see below), to the off-label use concerns of the FDA, and to the easy availability of methadone through community pharmacies and "script"-writing physicians.

The IND had in fact become a means for providing narcotic addiction treatment under the ostensible purpose of research. Although these IND-based treatment efforts, thinly disguised as research, resulted in annual reports that met FDA's IND reporting requirements for patient safety data, the protocols were not designed to obtain effectiveness data in support of an NDA and little attention was paid to the reports. (These treatment efforts did generate a large body of data on a large number of heroin addicts. The DNADA monitored the Cohen-IND investigators' reports for adverse effects of the drug, as did FDA for all INDs, but no effort was made by either agency to review and analyze the data systematically. The primary value of these data, when the 1972 FDA regulations were proposed and issued, was that they revealed no major negative consequences from treatment of addicts with methadone).

Even though the 1971 IND regulations were designed to permit the use of methadone for treatment of heroin addiction—under very strict federal controls—they were so restrictive that they discouraged its use. For example, the "acceptable protocol" that was to guide programs promoted rehabilitation and stipulated such measures of efficacy as arrest record, extent of alcohol abuse, extent of drug abuse, occupational adjustment, social adjustment, and "withdrawal from methadone and achievement of an enduring drug free status." In addition, the protocol also recommended that "initial dosage was to be low; for example, 20 milligrams per day," urinalyses were to be conducted weekly, and "participants who have maintained satisfactory adjustment over an extended period" were to be considered for discontinuation. Nevertheless, these 1971 regulations set the stage for 1972 FDA regulations that supplanted them.

1972 Regulations

New methadone regulations were proposed by FDA in April 1972 and issued in final form on December 15, 1972, (37 FR 26790). Although modified several times in the two decades since then, they established the basic DHHS framework that still exists for the regulation of methadone and constitutes the third layer of regulation, additional to the traditional approaches to regulation taken historically by the FDA and DEA (and its predecessors). The regulations removed methadone from general distribution and established controls over its use, literally on a patient by patient basis, through physician registration and treatment programs with characteristics prescribed in the regulations.

Two types of treatment—detoxification and maintenance—were defined. The former involved using methadone "as a substitute narcotic drug in decreasing doses to reach a drug free state in a period not to exceed 21 days" in order to "withdraw an individual who is dependent on heroin or other morphine-like drugs from the use of these drugs." Methadone maintenance, the provision of which was to be restricted to methadone treatment programs, involved using methadone "at relatively stable doses" for more than 21 days along with the appropriate social and medical services. The rule made it clear that although the goal of treatment was an "eventual drug free state," it differed from the 1971 regulation in the recognition "that for some patients the drug may be needed for long periods of time" (37 FR 26795, December 15, 1972).

In order to deny physicians, pharmacies, hospitals, or treatment programs the authority to prescribe, administer, or dispense methadone without prior approval by the FDA and the appropriate state agency, the regulations specified certain "organizational structures" as conditions of approval of participating programs. A two-tiered system was stipulated. The first tier—"methadone treatment programs"—provided comprehensive services using methadone for either detoxification or maintenance treatment of narcotic addicts, including initial patient evaluation. All facilities, hospitals, and outpatient units that conducted initial evaluations and dispensed the medication were considered separate programs, even though outpatient units might be part of a primary "centralized organizational structure." The second tier, a "methadone treatment medication units—referred to *a facility within a treatment program* that was "geographically dispersed" from the primary facility and other medical units and restricted to dispensing methadone and collecting urines to test for narcotic drugs.

Minimum program services, in addition to the dispensing of methadone, were to include counseling, rehabilitation, and other social services to help the patient "become a well functioning member of society." Programs not physically within a hospital were required to have formal agreements with some responsible hospital official to ensure that both inpatient and outpatient hospital care was fully available to any patient needing it. Neither the program sponsor nor the hospital was obligated to be financially responsible for such care. The regulation also required that individual physicians who wished to provide methadone treatment apply and be approved as a "program."

In order to operate a methadone treatment program, the regulation required simultaneous submission of an application to FDA and to the state authority for approval. In addition, before FDA approved a program it was to "first consult" with BNDD to determine compliance with the controlled substance law. Each specific physical site at which medication was to be dispensed required approval—for initial use or termination of use of methadone, or relocation of the site of use. Similarly, revocation of a program by a state authority required FDA revocation; FDA revocation required consultation with DEA.

Medication units were limited to 30 patients, referred by the primary unit who did not need the "frequent counseling, rehabilitative, and other services" of the primary facility and who had demonstrated "progress toward rehabilitation." Approval of medication units was by the FDA and the state authority based on the number of such units in a geographic area. The medication unit could receive its methadone supply only from the primary unit. Although revocation of a primary program's approval automatically revoked that of the medication unit, revocation of the latter did not have the opposite effect.

A program application required the name of the responsible individual, the location and responsibilities of each facility or medication unit, and all sources of funding for the program. Where two or more programs shared a central administration, as in a city- or state-wide organization, the responsible person was to be listed for each program. If an individual was medical director for more than one program, the feasibility of that arrangement had to be documented. Although sponsors were not required to be licensed physicians, they were required to employ a licensed physician as medical director. Those responsible for administering or dispensing the medication were "practitioners" as defined by the Controlled Substances Act and had to be licensed to practice in the state in which the program was established. The FDA and state authority were to be informed within three weeks of the replacement of a program sponsor or medical director.

A list of all hospitals, laboratories, and other related facilities providing comprehensive medical and rehabilitative services was required by FDA and the state authority. The application also required that the program estimate the "number of patients who will be treated, based on past history, addict population in the area, treatment capacity, or other relevant information."

Minimum admission standards, including voluntary consent to treatment, were set forth in detail. "Physiologic addiction standards" required that an individual patient be dependent on heroin for at least two years before being admitted to treatment, and the symptoms of withdrawal providing "evidence of physical dependence" are described in great detail. Patients under 16 years of age were precluded from treatment because the safety and effectiveness of treatment of adolescents had not been established, and special procedures were required for patients between 16 and 18 years of age. The contents of the patient evaluation and admission record were spelled out in detail with respect to the patient's personal history, medical history, and physician examination.

Methadone was to be administered orally (in liquid form) by treatment programs. Minimum dosage was described, both for detoxification treatment and for maintenance treatment. Initial recommended doses were limited to 15–20 mg, with 40 mg regarded usually an "adequate stabilizing dose." Stabilization was a two- or three-day period, after which doses could be reduced daily or every two days, the criterion being to "keep withdrawal symptoms at a tolerable level." Detoxification treatment longer than 3 weeks was seen as maintenance treatment.

For maintenance treatment for heavy users of heroin (i.e., those with tolerance), the initial dose should be adjusted to the individual's tolerance level; that dose could then be followed by 20 mg 4 to 8 hours later, or 40 mg in a single oral dose. If someone entered treatment with little or no tolerance, then doses in half these amounts were advised. Where doubt existed, the regulations indicated that the lower dose should prevail. Doses above 100 mg required that ingestion be observed six times a week. Doses above 120 mg required justification in the medical record and prior approval by the FDA and state authority. Take-home doses above 100 mg per day also required prior approval from the state authority and FDA. Physicians were encouraged to conduct a regular review of dosage with "careful consideration" given to its reduction. Methadone maintenance doses for pregnant patients were to be kept "as low as possible" if continued treatment was judged necessary.

Attendance for detoxification that required daily administration was to be "under close observation." Maintenance treatment was to be daily, or 6 times a week, for a minimum of 3 months. Then "after demonstrating satisfactory adherence to the program regulations for at least 3 months, and showing substantial progress in rehabilitation by participating actively in the program activities and/or by participation in educational, vocational, and homemaking activities, those patients whose employment, education, or homemaking responsibilities would be hindered by daily attendance" may be permitted to reduce observed medication taking to three times weekly and become eligible to receive no more than a two-day take-home supply. Documentation of progress and the need for reduced visits was required. Authorization to make exceptions for emergency responses—acute illness, family crisis, necessary travel—was provided.

The following provision of the rule (37 FR 26806) set forth the rationale for the FDA commissioner's action, and cited the need for data, the dangers of uncontrolled use, and the benefits of use:

> In view of the tremendous public health and social problems associated with the use of heroin, the demonstrated usefulness of methadone in treatment, the lack of a safe and effective alternative drug or treatment modality, the need for additional safety and effectiveness data on methadone and the danger to health that could be created by uncontrolled distribution and use of methadone, the Commissioner of Food and Drugs finds that it is not in the public interest either to withhold the drug from the market until it has been proved safe and effective under all conditions of use or to grant full approval for unrestricted distribution, prescription, dispensing, or administration of methadone. The Commissioner therefore concludes that it is essential to the public interest to prescribe detailed conditions for safe and effective use of methadone, utilizing the IND and NDA control mechanisms and the authority granted under the Comprehensive Drug Abuse Prevention and Control Act of 1970, to assure that the required additional information for assessing the safety and effectiveness of methadone is obtained, to maintain close control over the safe distribution, administration, and dispensing of the drug, and to detail responsibilities for such control.

The rule being promulgated was the vehicle for achieving these objectives.

Finally, to establish consistency with the new rule, the NDAs that had previously been issued to eight pharmaceutical firms for the use of methadone as an analgesic and antitussive, including Eli Lilly's original 1947 NDA, were withdrawn on the grounds that there was "a lack of substantial evidence that methadone is safe and effective for detoxification, analgesia, or antitussive use under the conditions of use that presently exist." The firms were granted opportunity for a hearing and invited to document with "a well-organized and full factual analysis of the data" a challenge to the basis for withdrawal and to submit a supplemental NDA "requesting approval for the manufacture and distribution of methadone" pursuant to the newly published rule. (See 37 FR 26807.)

The controlled distribution established by this rule restricted dispensing of methadone to hospital pharmacies and treatment programs, required registration of physicians, thus limiting their ability to write prescriptions for methadone for heroin addicts, and required that methadone treatment services be provided only by authorized programs. Some provisions of the rule became effective immediately; others on March 15, 1973.

Legal Challenge to the FDA

The closed distribution system authorized by this rule restricted methadone use for analgesic purposes to hospital pharmacies. This basically removed methadone from most retail pharmacies, reversing a situation that had existed since 1947. Insulted, and perhaps fearing additional restrictions on the professional practice of pharmacy, the American Pharmaceutical Association, which represents the pharmacy profession, successfully challenged this portion of the FDA rule in 1974 in *APhA v. Weinberger* (377 F. Suppl. 824, D.D.C., 1974). The U.S. District Court for the District of Columbia held that FDA lacked statutory authority to impose certain postapproval controls on methadone and, therefore, that methadone could be marketed and distributed through retail pharmacies like any other schedule II narcotic. In 1976, the U.S. Court of Appeals upheld the lower court (*APhA v. Mathews*, 530 F.2d 1054, 1976), and broadened its prohibition against postapproval controls. An FDA request for Supreme Court review was denied by the Department of Justice. The result was that FDA amended its regulations in July 1976 (41 FR 28262) to allow general dispensing of methadone for analgesia but to continue its restricted distribution for narcotic addiction treatment.

Narcotic Addict Treatment Act of 1974

The final piece of the legal framework for regulating the use of methadone for treating narcotic addiction was the adoption of the Narcotic Addict Treatment Act (NATA) of 1974 (Public Law 93-281), which amended the Controlled Substances Act. This legislation was driven by concern for the diversion of methadone to illicit channels that was occurring in 1972 and 1973, as reflected in the title of the Senate bill adopted on June 8, 1973, the Methadone Diversion Control Act of 1973. (U.S. Senate, 1970a, 1970b).

The Subcommittee to Investigate Juvenile Delinquency of the Senate Committee on the Judiciary held hearings on methadone diversion on November 14 and 16, 1972, and February 8, 13, and 14, and April 5, 1973. As the FDA regulations became effective only on March 15, 1973, the work of the Senate had largely been done by that time. The Judiciary Committee report cited a number of instances of physicians writing methadone prescriptions at a very high rate and making substantial monies in the process. The House acted on March 19, 1974, changing the bill title to that which was enacted by the whole Congress. The bill was signed into law on May 14, 1974.

The legislative history of NATA makes clear that the regulations and the statute were seen as complementary. In the Senate hearings on the bill, Dr. John Jennings, associate commissioner for medical affairs of FDA, testified: "We feel that this bill will, in a way, complement the regulations that the FDA have [sic] developed jointly with the Justice Department and other agencies. It will not replace them in any way; it will simply make their enforcement much more readily obtainable." The purpose of the bill, the Senate committee report stated, was "to provide new authority for the regulation of the use of narcotic drugs in the treatment of narcotic addicts which are consistent with legitimate program objectives and the protection of the community at large." The House report expressed the belief that the bill would "complement the DEA and FDA regulations currently in force, and establish the basis for additional joint regulation of treatment programs by these two agencies." The intent of Congress was clear on the expectation that the law would be implemented by regulations.

As had the methadone regulation, the NATA statute defined both maintenance and detoxification treatment. Maintenance treatment involved the "dispensing, for a period in excess of twenty-one days, of a narcotic drug in the treatment of an individual for dependence upon heroin or other morphine-like drugs." "Detoxification treatment" involved dispensing for less than 21 days, in decreasing doses sufficient to prevent withdrawal symptoms, "as a method of bringing the individual to a drug free state."

The act required a separate annual registration with DEA for practitioners dispensing methadone for either type of treatment. It was at this pint that the statutory role of the Secretary of HHS (then HEW) was established: The act stipulated that the Attorney General "shall register an applicant" (i.e., approve an application) meeting these criteria: (1) the applicant is determined "by the Secretary to be qualified (under standards established by the Secretary) to engage in the treatment" for which registration is sought; (2) the Attorney General determines that the applicant will comply with standards set by the Attorney General regarding the security of stocks of narcotic drugs and the maintenance of records on such drugs; and (3) the Secretary determines the applicant will comply with standards set by the Secretary (after consultation with the Attorney General) "respecting the quantities of narcotic drugs which may be provided for unsupervised use by individuals in such treatment." In addition, the Attorney General was authorized to revoke or suspend immediately the registration of any practitioner not meeting the standards of the act.

Summary: 1970–1974

During the five-year period from 1970 through 1974, an extensive regulatory framework was established for the use of methadone in the treatment of narcotic addiction. Authority of the Secretary (originally of HEW, now of HHS) to issue standards of treatment for narcotic addiction treatment, specifically for the qualifications of practitioners and with respect to the quantities of methadone for take-home ("unsupervised use"), was embedded in the NATA provision for registration of practitioners by DEA. This statute, in turn, reinforced the authority previously articulated in the 1972 regulations issued by FDA. DEA authority was established under the Controlled Substances Act, primarily in the NATA amendments to that act, regarding the registration of applicants meeting specific criteria, some of which were determined by the Attorney General and some by the Secretary, and the security of stocks of narcotic medications and the associated record keeping.

In the words of the Senate Committee report, there was now "new authority" to regulate treatment programs; in the words of the House Committee report, there was now "the basis for additional joint regulation" by FDA and DEA. With the Secretary of HHS obligated to assure standards of treatment, the "third layer" was now in place.

THE CURRENT REGULATORY REGIME

1980 Revision of the Regulations

In 1980, the methadone regulations were revised, partly in response to the 1974 NATA. The revision was based on two notices of proposed rule-making, the first issued by FDA (41 FR 17926, April 29, 1976), and the second issued jointly by FDA and NIDA (42 FR 56897, October 28, 1977). The changes might be described as "fine-tuning" and not an alteration of the fundamental scheme.

The 1980 final rule (45 FR 62694, September 19, 1980) reduced the minimum standard for admission from two years of addiction to one year coupled with a clinical determination that the individual was currently physiologically dependent. Exceptions were made for four groups. First, persons in penal or chronic care institutions were allowed to enroll in a treatment program as early as 14 days before release and as late as six months after release; previously, the period had ranged from 7 days before to 7 days after release. Second, pregnant women addicts, for whom the risk of return to illicit narcotic use was judged greater than the risk of methadone, were also exempted, with the requirement that they be examined within three months after termination of pregnancy regarding the appropriate treatment course. Third, previously treated maintenance patients who had voluntarily detoxified were also exempted from the one-year requirement for admission; in essence, they were not required to return to illicit drug use before being readmitted to a program. Finally, persons under 16 years of age were now admissible to maintenance treatment; previously only detoxification had been allowed.

The rule retained mandatory urine testing for methadone maintenance patients of at least eight tests in the first year of treatment, at least quarterly tests for the second and successive years, and monthly tests for each six-day take-home patient. This represented a trade-off between the need to control diversion, a regard for practitioners costs, and a concern to avoid interfering in the physician-patient relationship. The rule stated that states were free to impose more stringent testing requirements if they chose.

The evaluation of a patient in an admission interview could now be conducted by a well-trained program counselor, not necessarily a mental health professional.

The final rule recommended but did not require that programs not providing required services on-site document formal agreements with other providers of these services. Neither "program services" nor "comprehensive rehabilitative services" were defined in terms of the variable needs of individual patients.

The medical director and other program physicians were to be licensed to practice medicine in the jurisdiction in which the program was located. The minimum staffing patterns section did not define the minimum qualifications for counselors nor provide a definition of a methadone counselor, leaving such matters to program administrators. A minimum ratio of one counselor to 50 patients was required, which could be met by a combination of full- or part-time personnel.

The initial dosage was limited to 30 mg per day, with an additional 10 mg allowable in the 4 to 8 hours after initial administration if needed to suppress withdrawal symptoms. Although comments to the proposed rule had challenged setting the dosage for pregnant addicts as low as possible, this provision was retained in the final rule, thus balancing "desire to treat the mother effectively and [desire] to protect the fetus from potential adverse effects." The usual range of maintenance doses in 1980 was between 40 and 100 mg. Doses over 100 mg required that the state authority and the FDA be notified in writing or by telephone within 72 hours of the dose, eliminating the requirement of prior approval.

The final rule restricted take-home methadone to a liquid form for "responsible" patients. The decision was to be made or reviewed by a physician, usually after consulting appropriate staff, using these criteria: absence of recent abuse of drugs; regularity of clinic attendance; absence of serious behavioral problems at the clinic; absence of known criminal activity; stability of patient's home environment and social relationships; length of time in maintenance treatment; assurance of safe storage at home; potential risks of diversion were outweigh by the rehabilitative benefit of decreasing the frequency of clinic attendance.

Take-home medication was allowed after daily observation (or at least observation on six days a week) in the first three months of treatment; then the patient could receive two-day take-homes for the next two years in treatment; finally, conditional on good behavior, three-day take-homes were authorized. If good behavior was observed for three treatment years, a weekly take-home of six-days was allowed. Restriction or probationary withdrawal of take-home privileges was required if scheduled clinic appointments were missed, or if a urine test was positive for morphine-like drugs or negative for methadone. Take-homes were not permitted for patients with a daily dose greater than 100 mg.

For detoxification, the standard was defined as 21 days or less of treatment, consistent with the NATA. (The preamble noted that this statutory definition could not be changed by regulation, but maintained that detoxification requiring longer than 21 days' treatment "may easily be accomplished" within the regulatory framework "as long as a patient met maintenance treatment criteria (45 FR 62705).) No take-homes were allowed; the recommended initial dose was between 15 and 20 mg; and at least one week was required between successive detoxification efforts.

Hospital use of methadone for patients admitted for narcotic addiction treatment was limited to three weeks; longer treatment could be provided only in a maintenance program. A maintenance patient hospitalized for the treatment of medical conditions other than narcotic addiction and requiring "temporary maintenance treatment" during his or her stay could receive maintenance treatment.

1989 Revision of the Regulations

The regulations were next revised in 1989, following two proposals to modify them, one in 1983 and one in 1987.

1983 Regulatory Reform Initiative

Under President Ronald Reagan, a government-wide effort was made to review all federal government regulations and to eliminate or reduce the burden of these regulations on the private sector, state and local governments, and nonprofit organizations. This general effort prompted a review of the methadone regulations in 1983. The review team recommended the following:

- With the exception of the take-home requirements and certain application and admission criteria (not identified), the methadone regulations should be basically in the form of guidelines.
- Certification to the Drug Enforcement Administration that treatment standards are met should be made after an on-site inspection is conducted.
- On-site inspections should be conducted annually for each treatment program for purposes of enforcing or ensuring/compliance with the treatment standards.

In transmitting the results of the review, the chairman of the review team cautioned that while all review team members concurred with the recommendations, the effort to select specific regulations for conversion to guidelines would reveal "unresolved policy issues."

The 1983 review argued the case for guidelines on the following basis:

> Since 1972 when the first methadone regulations were issued and continuing into the present, the "state of the art" in the treatment and rehabilitation of narcotic addicts has been evolving and frequently changing. An often voiced criticism of

the Federal regulations is that changes in the regulations have not kept pace with the "state of the art" and are too inflexible to allow adequate treatment.

An example of the slow adaptation cited was the discrepancy between the detoxification limit of 21 days in the 1980 regulation and the results of the "latest research data" (in 1983) that showed the need for up to 180 days for rehabilitation to occur.

The report distinguished three DHHS regulatory functions: standards, certification, and enforcement/compliance. The options for standards were regulations, guidelines, or labeling; for certification the options were DHHS certification to DEA, DHHS inspectional authority, pro forma reliance on states, or written commitment by practitioners; for enforcement and compliance, the options were on-site inspection or none at all.

The review team concluded that "the current approach" of regulations was adequate for certification and enforcement/compliance. Regarding standards, the review team reached consensus on the following:

> that most aspects of the current methadone standards (with the take-home requirements and certain application and admission criteria in the regulations the primary exceptions) should be changed from regulations to guidelines and that the reduction in the level of detailed regulation would not seriously adversely affect the quality and level of treatment to patients enrolled in narcotic addict treatment programs.

The report noted that DEA staff had, informally, raised no objections to the recommended approach "as long as diversion does not increase." Thus, the review team recommended that the DHHS treatment standards "be basically in the form of guidelines."

In response to this exercise, in 1983, the FDA and NIDA solicited comment on whether they should make portions of the methadone regulation into guidelines, and modify record-keeping and reporting requirements, and whether changing the requirements "would impair enforcement and compliance with the regulation, affect the quality of patient care, and increase the likelihood of the diversion of methadone for illicit use." Most of the comments viewed the methadone regulations as "generally neither unreasonable nor burdensome" and most argued that they should not be substantially revised or converted to guidelines.

1987 Notice of Proposed Rule-Making

The 1983 recommendations, though not adopted, did initiate another revision of the methadone regulations, which first found expression in a 1987 proposed rule (52 FR 37047, October 2, 1987) and culminated in a final rule (54 FR 8954, March 2, 1989) at the end of the decade. In the 1987 proposed rule, the FDA and NIDA, in an effort to put the best face on the unenthusiastic 1983 response by the provider community to converting the regulations to guidelines, indicated that they had retained the "current requirements necessary to achieve the goals" of the 1974 NATA, but were proposing to "streamline" the regulation and to "promote more efficient operation of methadone programs."

The most significant revision proposed was to develop separate guidelines "consisting of those provisions of the current regulation that are not legal requirements." Therefore, language beginning with "It is recommended practice that" was to be dropped from the regulation and incorporated into an accompanying guidance document.

The 1987 proposed rule, issued by the FDA and NIDA, advanced the following changes in the methadone regulation: that detoxification treatment be divided into short-term (<21 days) and long-term (>21 and <180 days) treatment; that the minimum staffing ratio of one counselor to 50 patients be eliminated; that blood tests be allowed as ways to conduct initial drug screening or to meet the monthly testing requirements for six-day take-home patients; that the 72-hour notification of FDA and the pertinent state authority for methadone doses greater than 100 mg be eliminated; that special adverse reaction reporting requirements for methadone be eliminated and reliance placed upon general FDA reporting requirements; that a supervising counselor be allowed to conduct the annual review of the patient's treatment plan for "certain qualified patients" who had been in treatment for 3 years or longer; and that the requirement of an annual report of methadone treatment programs to the FDA be dropped.

The agencies rejected the option that the federal government rely exclusively on state and local regulations. Federal involvement was required by NATA to "ensure that only bona fide narcotic addicts" were admitted to treatment, "to limit the potential for illicit diversion," and to set forth "minimum standards for the treatment of narcotic addicts with methadone." However, throughout the proposal, FDA and NIDA proposed to defer to the judgment of treatment programs and to leave to state and local governments the responsibility for stricter regulation. The summary noted that authority existed for the federal government to contract with states for inspection and compliance with the federal regulations. The suggestion that the federal government rely on the (then) Joint Commission on the Accreditation of Hospitals and its alcohol guideline was rejected as inappropriate to drug abuse.

1989 Final Rule

The FDA and NIDA issued a final rule on March 2, 1989, based on comments on the 1987 proposed (54 FR 8954). Although the rule modified the methadone regulations somewhat, it left the fundamental structure intact. The major changes to the regulations as issued in 1980 included the following: detoxification was separated into short- and long-term, the former being a maximum of 30 days and the latter a maximum of 180 days; a specified counselor-patient ratio was deleted; treatment programs were allowed to use other procedures besides urinalysis, such as blood testing, to test for drugs of abuse; the 72-hour notification of FDA and state authority for doses above 100 mg was eliminated, but written justification in the patient record was still required; the review of a patient's annual treatment plan by a physician was not required for model patients in treatment for 3 years; the serology test for syphilis could be omitted if a patient's veins were so severely damaged as to preclude obtaining blood; expanded counseling for pregnant women was required; an inadvertently omitted requirement that a physician date and sign the patient record within 72 hours of first administration of methadone was reinstated; and the special adverse reaction reporting requirement for methadone and the annual report to FDA were eliminated.

Some provider comments on the 1987 proposed rule reflected a fear that removal of rehabilitation services requirements would weaken the emphasis on rehabilitation. The agencies' response was that they believed "that a program's staff is in the best position to determine what services are needed" (54 FR 8956, March 2, 1989). A suggestion that the roles of physicians, counseling directors, and counselors be clearly delineated evoked the response that the regulation's purpose, as defined by NATA, was "to develop "appropriate methods of professional practice in the *medical* treatment" of narcotic addiction. Similarly, the response to a request for criteria differentiating between short- and long-term detoxification left that judgment with the treatment program.

On the other hand, the FDA and NIDA rejected a suggestion that the requirement for 6-days per week observation of a patient receiving greater than 100 mg of methadone represented interference in the professional judgment of a physician for which there was "no medical justification." Rather, the agencies held that such doses "present a high risk of diversion" and that "concerns about the possibility of diversion must outweigh concerns about infringing on the clinical judgment of the program's physician" (54 FR 8959).

1989 Guidance Document

Concurrently, FDA and NIDA issued a six-page guidance document, which noted that the regulations, over time, had recommended "certain practices" that were not actually required. The document was consolidating these recommended practices (the "shoulds") for medical and other services for the treatment of narcotic addicts; the requirements (the "shalls") were retained in the regulations. The guidance document dealt with services; hospital affiliation; medication units; current physiological dependence; drug screening urinalysis; contents of medical evaluation; admission evaluation; initial treatment plans and their periodic evaluation; pregnant patients, staffing; and initial, maintenance, take-home, and initial detoxification dosage; methadone formulation; and discontinuation of methadone use (both involuntary and voluntary).

The document stated that "medical services and counseling, rehabilitative, and other social services" should normally be available at the primary outpatient facility but might be provided under contract with other organizations, either on-site or elsewhere. If not physically within a hospital, a formal agreement should exist indicating that hospital care, including emergency, inpatient, and ambulatory care, is "fully available" to any patient needing it. Medication units should serve a geographic area separate and distinct from the primary facility and of "reasonable size" relative to the treatment space.

In determining "current physiological dependence," the report advised physicians to consider both signs and symptoms of intoxication and early signs of withdrawal.

In the use of urinalysis for program decisions, the guidance document advised programs to "show evidence of reasonable confirmatory laboratory analysis." Urinalysis was described as "one clinical tool" for diagnosis and making treatment plans and "one technique" for program evaluation by monitoring pre- and posttreatment drug use patterns. The document stated that "a person could be currently dependent on narcotic drugs without having a positive urine test for narcotics [i.e., could produce a false negative]," or a person "could have a positive urine test for narcotics and not be currently physiologically dependent [i.e., could produce a false positive]," and thus testing should not be used as the exclusive basis for admission for treatment.

The contents of the medical evaluation were specified in detail. The acquisition of information about a patient's psychosocial, economic, and family background that revealed "strengths and weaknesses" was left to individual programs.

Dosage was spelled out for initiation of treatment (15–30 mg for heavy users of heroin, with lesser amounts 4 to 8 hours later; one-half these amounts for those with "little or no tolerance"), and the range of maintenance was indicated as between 40 mg and 100 mg daily.

1989 Interim Methadone Maintenance Proposal

On March 2, 1989, simultaneously with publication of the revision of the regulations and the issuance of the guidance document, two other actions were taken by FDA and NIDA: a proposed rule was issued on interim methadone maintenance; and comment was solicited on a pilot study on "improved measures of methadone performance."

Interim methadone maintenance was a variation from established methadone practice, by which methadone, but no other services, could be provided on a temporary basis to addicted persons for whom treatment slots were available; it was being proposed by the FDA and NIDA "in response to the HIV epidemic in the intravenous (IV) drug abusing population" and was "intended to help reduce the spread of HIV infection" (54 FR 8973, March 2, 1989). HIV was "making massive inroads" among intervenous drug users; methadone treatment, by reducing the consumption of heroin by needle sharing, could therefore reduce the spread of HIV.[6]

Under the proposal, methadone maintenance treatment was to be categorized as "comprehensive" and "interim." The former was methadone maintenance treatment as defined in the existing regulations. Although "interim" treatment was to be provided only by comprehensive treatment programs (i.e., programs offering only interim treatment were prohibited), it was intended to give programs the flexibility to "dispense methadone to medically evaluated narcotic addicts who are awaiting placement in comprehensive maintenance treatment."

Programs would be required to provide a medical examination and service, but not rehabilitative services. They would also be required to "counsel patients on reducing the risk of HIV-transmission." Methadone would have to be ingested under observation; therefore, random drug screening tests would be not be required. Take-home medication would be prohibited, so clinics would have to be open seven days a week. The initial treatment plan and periodic plan evaluation required of "comprehensive" programs would not be

---

[6]The proposal arose from increased concern within the Public Health Service about the general HIV epidemic and the increasing spread of HIV to intravenous drug users. In addition, a study at Beth Israel Medical Center, New York, funded by the Centers for Disease Control, showed methadone to be effective in reducing needle use among methadone patients.

required for "interim" treatment. Nor would the assignment of a primary counselor to a patient be required.

Under the proposal, programs would be required "to establish and follow reasonable written priorities, which may take into account medical and rehabilitative factors, for transferring patients from interim maintenance treatment to comprehensive maintenance treatment." Transfer was anticipated by FDA and NIDA after "a relatively brief period," but no times were specified for such transfer. However, if a patient was continued in interim treatment for six months, a formal evaluation would be required to see "how the patient meets the transfer priority criteria."

In general, response to the "interim" maintenance proposal rule was strongly negative, especially by providers and state methadone authorities, although the American Medical Association was supportive. In April the FDA and NIDA extended the initial comment period until May 3, 1989. On December 4, they announced a public hearing for February 28, 1990, and extended the comment period an additional 15 days beyond the hearing (54 FR 50226).

Twenty-eight individuals, representing 20 organizations, testified at the hearing. Most of the comment was negative. The evidence on waiting lists showed some regional shortages but did not support a national capacity shortage. Moreover, it was argued that an *exemption* process at FDA permitted a treatment program to apply for and receive approval to conduct the equivalent of an interim maintenance treatment program, making the proposal unnecessary. The polydrug use of injecting narcotic addicts argued for the counseling and rehabilitative services of a comprehensive program.

Importantly, it was pointed out that the resources available to such programs would be reduced if treatment programs also devoted funds to interim maintenance. Providers also feared that providing interim treatment at reduced costs per patient would lead policymakers to reduce their per slot budget allocations for maintenance patients. In light of these factors, many concluded that the proposal would fail in its objective.

On May 23, 1990, therefore, the director of NIDA informed his superiors "that today the PHS Methadone Work Group agreed to begin the formal process to rescind the proposal of March 2, 1989." Only the requirement of counseling "on avoidance and transmission" of HIV was to be issued, which would apply to both maintenance and detoxification treatment.

Independently of the proposed "interim" methadone regulation, however, efforts were underway within the Public Health Service, in Congress, and elsewhere, to reorganize the Alcohol, Drug Abuse, and Mental Health Administration (ADAMHA). These efforts culminated in the ADAMHA Reorganization Act of 1992 (Public Law 102-321, July 10, 1992), the main purpose of which was to transfer the research portions of the three ADAMHA institutes—NIDA, the National Institute of Alcoholism and Alcohol Abuse, and the National Institute of Mental Health—to the National Institutes of Health and to create the Substance Abuse and Mental Health Services Administration (SAMHSA) as the home for the service functions of these entitles.

However, a secondary provision of the 1992 Act, introduced as an amendment to the House bill by Rep. Henry Waxman, gave a statutory basis to interim maintenance, thus blocking the effort that HHS had begun to rescind its proposed rule of 1989. Consequently, on January 6, 1993, regulations were issued implementing this provision (58 FR 495).[7] As of 1994, no treatment program had chosen to implement the optional provisions of the interim methadone maintenance rule other than the requirement of HIV counseling.

Assessment of Program Performance

Also on March 2, 1989, an advance notice was published (54 FR 8976), which solicited comments on a pilot study "designed to help identify improved measures of methadone program performance and thus enhance the quality of treatment." Subsequently, a Request for Proposals was issued and a contract for the Methadone Treatment Quality Assurance Feasibility Study (MTQAS) was awarded to the Research Triangle Institute of North Carolina. The purpose of this study is to determine the feasibility of developing a performance-based reporting and feedback system and to evaluate how performance-based monitoring might be used to modify the current regulatory structure for methadone.

LEVO-ALPHA-ACETYL-METHADOL

On July 20, 1993, the FDA and NIDA issued an interim rule (58 FR 38704), effective immediately, with 60 days for public comment, which revised the methadone regulation to provide standards for the use of levo-alpha-acetyl-methadol (LAAM) in the maintenance treatment of narcotic addicts. Simultaneously, the FDA was approving an NDA for LAAM.[8]

---

[7]This rule was issued jointly by the FDA and SAMHSA.

[8]LAAM had been developed originally in 1948 as a synthetic congener of methadone, had been tested in Germany as a narcotic analgesic, and had been examined in this country as a potential narcotic addiction treatment medication in the 1970s. Consideration had languished in the 1980s until the Anti-Drug Abuse Act of 1988 (Public Law 100-690) authorized an expanded drug development effort within NIDA. The newly formed NIDA Medications Development Program then took the leadership

The interim rule noted that the 1989 revision of the methadone regulation had anticipated the approval of other drugs besides methadone for narcotic addiction treatment by changing many methadone-specific terms to general narcotic treatment drug terms. The interim rule reorganized the methadone regulation into three sections: general requirements that applied to all narcotic treatment programs regardless of the drug used; specific requirements applicable to LAAM; and specific requirements for methadone.

In one sense, the LAAM interim rule, with its three-part division (general, LAAM, and methadone) represents the evolution of the methadone regulation into a framework that is able to accept additional medications by the simple addition of new sections and appropriate paragraphs. In another sense, however, it represents the dominance of the beliefs that formed the underpinning of the methadone regulations over fresh thinking about the appropriateness for other antinarcotic medications that are themselves narcotics.

The interim rule did revise 21 CFR 291.501, basically unchanged since 1972, which had served as the defacto "preamble" to the methadone regulation.[9] The "need for further research" language, which had provided the justification for the hybrid IND-NDA system, was finally replaced by an explicit recognition by the FDA, NIDA, and DEA "that the use of narcotic drugs in the prolonged maintenance of narcotic dependence has been shown to be an effective part of a total treatment effort in the management and rehabilitation of selected narcotic addicts."[10]

The new section 291.501 noted the dangers of abuse if services and controls were inadequately applied. However, it simply indicated that interested professionals, municipalities, and organizations "should be allowed to use narcotic drugs in the medical treatment of narcotic addiction within a framework of adequate controls designed to protect the individual patients and the community."

The interim rule included the following LAAM-related provisions: take-home medications were prohibited; programs were prohibited from admitting individuals into treatment who were under 18 years of age; women of child-

---

in securing its approval as an NDA.

[9]This section of the 1972 regulations had been slightly changed in 1977.

[10]Although the need for "more research" was a legal justification for the hybrid 1972 IND-NDA regulation, it was used politically to resist public approval of methadone treatment as late as the 1988 White House Conference for a Drug Free America. Although the report of that conference recommended that treatment capacity be increased for "a full range of treatment approaches," including self-help groups, short-term treatment (both inpatient and outpatient), and long-term residential care, it also proposed that an independent organization evaluate the efficacy of methadone treatment.

bearing age seeking treatment were required to have a *monthly* pregnancy test; patients could not receive the medication more often than every other day at doses, frequencies, and under conditions of use prescribed in the approved labeling; for a previously stabilized methadone patient, initial doses were to be 1.3 times the daily methadone dose, not to exceed 120 mg of LAAM; a licensed physician was required to assume responsibility for the amount of drug dispensed and for recording changes in dosage in the patient's record; the drug was to be dispensed in liquid form, with a taste and color distinguishable from methadone.

The NDA for LAAM was approved by FDA on July 9, 1993 and LAAM was then rescheduled from a schedule I controlled substance to a schedule II substance (58 FR 43795, August 18, 1993). Comments on the interim rule challenged the assertion that treatment capacity would be increased by the longer duration of LAAM, criticized the prohibition on take-homes, sought clarification on dosage in relation to methadone doses, questioned the need for monthly pregnancy testing on grounds of costs, asked whether methadone treatment programs would be automatically approved to use LAAM, and complained that the FDA-approved label had not been published with the rule. California proprietary providers objected to the requirement that a physician complete and record initial patient evaluation findings *before* administering the medication, preferring that the physician either sign in advance or review the decision of a "health professional" within 72 hours of initial dose.

Whatever the limits imposed on LAAM by the federal methadone regulations, the implementation of LAAM regulation revealed that state regulations of the use of narcotics for the treatment of narcotic addiction were generally more constraining. In a memorandum of November 4, 1993, addressed to Dr. Frank Vocci, of the NIDA Medications Development Program, H. Alex Bradford, Chief Executive Officer of the BioDevelopment Corporation, the commercial sponsor of LAAM, outlined the complexity of the state approval process. He identified "five general areas" that needed to be addressed before an individual clinic (i.e., treatment program) could purchase LAAM:

1. Existing state treatment regulations, which covered methadone, needed to be modified for LAAM, which in many states required legislation unless an interim administrative process was employed.

2. The rescheduling of LAAM (as a controlled substance) was required in many states.

3. The addition of LAAM to the state formulary of medications approved for treating opiate dependence was required.

4. LAAM needed to be included in the list of reimbursable medications for treating opioid dependence.

5. The approval of LAAM's use in the clinic by county and local organizations having responsibility for overseeing the treatment clinics in their jurisdiction was often required.

The Bradford memorandum opens a window onto state regulation of the use of narcotics for narcotic addiction that shows that it is very extensive and considerably more variable than federal regulation. Viewed historically, state regulation is far more developed today than it was when methadone was initially approved by FDA.

SUMMARY

Although there has been some evolution and refinement, the methadone (and now LAAM) regulations in 1994 are fundamentally based on several assumptions that led to their issuance in 1972:

1. That use of a narcotic drug to treat narcotic addiction is an unusual practice posing special risks to patients, both those truly addicted and those who might be more appropriately treated without narcotic drugs;
2. That the desirability and availability of methadone created an unusual potential for drug diversion to illicit uses, posing special risks to society (see chapter 4);
3. That the regulatory controls imposed by the Federal Food, Drug, and Cosmetic Act and the Controlled Substances Act, as well as by state and local laws, on all other therapeutic drugs that also have a potential for abuse are inadequate to protect patients and society from these special risks; and
4. That a third set of federal regulations, thrusting FDA into a direct role of overseeing medical practice on a patient-by-patient basis, is necessary to assure protection.

In the course of its deliberations, the committee concluded that these assumptions are flawed and must be reexamined by HHS. Prior reviews of the regulations, proposed rules, final rules, guidelines, and public discussion have questioned these assumptions to some extent, but the comprehensive and public reevaluation of them has yet to take place. Although the committee does support some continued special regulation of methadone, it finds many of the current requirements excessively intrusive into medical practice, inimical to proper patient care and public health, and unnecessary to protect public safety as specified in chapters 7 and 8.

REFERENCES

Besteman, K. (1992). Federal Leadership in Building the National Drug Treatment System, Institute of Medicine. *Treating Drug Problems*, Vol. 2, Gertein, DR and Harwood, HJ, eds. National Academy Press, Washington, D.C.

Center for Drug Evaluation and Research of the Food and Drug Administration and the National Institute on Drug Abuse. 1989. Guidance on the Use of Methadone in Maintenance and Detoxification Treatment of Narcotic Addicts. March.

Conversation with Vincent Dole. 1994. *Addiction* (89):23–29.

Dole, VP, and Nyswander, M. 1965. A medical treatment for diacetylmorphine (heroin) addiction. *Journal of the American Medical Association* 193:80–84

Dole, VP, Nyswander, ME, and Kreek, MJ. 1966. Narcotic blockade: A medical technique for stopping heroin use by addicts. *Transactions of the Association of American Physicians* 79:122–136.

Dole, VP. (1989). In Courtwright, D, Joseph, H, Des Jarlais, D, *Addicts Who Survived: An Oral History of Narcotic Use in America, 1923–1965*, Knoxville, University of Tennessee Press 331–343.

Draft Final Rule, Food and Drug Administration, National Institute of Drug Abuse, "Methadone in maintenance and detoxification treatment of narcotic addicts; human immunodeficiency virus counseling," unpublished, n.d.

Institute of Medicine. 1991. Research and Service Programs in the PHS: Challenges in Organization. Washington, D.C., National Academy Press.

Letters to the FDA Dockets Management Branch from the following: Nina Peyser, Executive Director, Chemical Dependency Institute, Beth Israel Medical Center, New York, NY, August 24, 1994; Forest Tennant, MD, Dr.PH, Community Health Projects Medical Group, West Covina, Calif., September 7, 1993; James L. Sorensen, Ph.D., Chief, Substance Abuse Services, San Francisco General Hospital, San Francisco, Calif., September 14, 1993; Frank McGurk, Chairperson, New York Committee of Methadone Program Administrators, New York, NY, September 15, 1993; Melvin Sabshin, M.D., Medical Director, American Psychiatric Association, Washington, D.C., September 22, 1993; and Andrew M. Mecca, Dr.P.H., Director, Department of Alcohol and Drug Programs, State of California-Health and Welfare Agency, Sacramento, Calif., September 27, 1993.

Letters to FDA Dockets Management Branch from the following: Kenneth Teruya Akinaka, M.R.A., Quality Improvement Coordinator, Bay Area Addiction Research and Treatment, San Francisco, Calif., 9/14/93; and Robert B. Kahn, Ph.D., President, California Organization of Methadone Providers, San Diego, Calif., September 23, 1993.

Memorandum to Dr. John Gregrich, ONDCP, Mr. Chris Petula, Senate Judiciary Committee, Ms. Denise Courier, Drug Enforcement Administration, and Dr. Frank Vocci, Medications Development Division, NIDA, from H. Alex Bradford, CEO, BioDevelopment Corporation, November 4, 1993.

Memorandum to Chairman, Methadone Retrospective Review Team, from Peter H. Reinstein, M.D., Acting Director, Office of Drugs, Food and Drug Administration, re "Revised Final Report—Retrospective Review of Methadone Regulations," September 9, 1983.

Memorandum to Chairman, Retrospective Review Committee, from Edwin V. Dutra, Jr., Chairman, re "Methadone Retrospective Review of the Methadone Regulations," August 26, 1983.

Memorandum from Charles R. Schuster, Director, NIDA, to Dr. Frederick Goodwin, Administrator, Alcohol, Drug Abuse, and Mental Health Administration, Mr. Mark Barnes, Counsel to the Secretary, Dr. James Mason, Assistant Secretary for Health, and Dr. Herbert Kleber, Office of National Drug Control Policy, "Federal Methadone Regulation—Proposed Revision to Allow Interim Treatment," May 23, 1990.

Nightingale, SL. 1993. Associate Commissioner for Health Affairs, Food and Drug Administration, letter to Richard A. Rettig, Ph.D. (June 21).

Revisions to the Federal Methadone Regulation (21 CFR 291.505), document provided by National Institute of Drug Abuse, n.d.

U.S. Senate, Committee on Judiciary. 1973a. *Narcotic Addict Treatment Act* Hearings, 93rd Congress, 1st Session (April 5). p. 697

U.S. Senate, Committee on the Judiciary. 1973b. *Methadone Diversion Control Act* Report No. 93-192, 93rd Congress, 1st Session (June 4).

U.S. House of Representatives, Interstate and Foreign Commerce Committee. 1970. Comprehensive Drug Abuse Prevention and Control Act of 1970 Report No. 91-1444, 91st Congress, 2nd Session (September 10).

U.S. House of Representatives, Interstate and Foreign Commerce Committee. 1974. *Narcotic Addict Treatment Act* Report No. 93-884, 93rd Congress, 2nd Session (March 7).

Yancowitz SR, Des Jarlais DC, Peyser NP, Drew E, Friedmann P, Trigg HL, and Robinson JW. A randomized trial of an interim methadone maintenance clinic. Am J Public Health 81:1185–1191, September 1991.

6

Methadone Treatment

This chapter describes the characteristics of methadone treatment providers, the financing of treatment, and how several states with large addict populations regulate and finance treatment. It draws on several data bases, each of which has certain limitations. These limits are discussed below as appropriate.

THE PROVIDER COMMUNITY

This section describes the characteristics of providers of outpatient methadone maintenance programs—the number of treatment facilities, the regional distribution of facilities, the number of patients, and the capacity, utilization, waiting time, and ownership.

Methadone is used currently to treat opiate addiction by detoxification and maintenance. Detoxification treatment accounts for 8 percent of all methadone patients nationally (Batten et al, 1993), but for a much higher percentage in California (see below and chapter 3). Methadone maintenance treatment is normally provided by an outpatient treatment program. Programs have four common features: a dispensing unit, counseling offices, examining rooms, and an administrative area (Ball and Ross, 1991). They often vary with regard to methadone dosing, take-home policies, and other treatment factors (General Accounting Office, 1990; Ball and Ross, 1991; D'Aunno and Vaughn, 1992). In addition to dispensing medication, programs also provide counseling and other medical services.

Number of Treatment Facilities

FDA, in its 1994 registry of programs approved to dispense methadone under the Narcotic Addict Treatment Act, documents 780 active programs app-

151

roved for methadone maintenance and 275 approved for detoxification in calendar year 1993 (Food and Drug Administration, 1993; E. Dory, FDA, personal communication, 1994). The data on maintenance programs may overestimate the total: FDA counts as a "program" an individual dispensing site, and large programs often may have more than one site; and once approved by FDA, a program remains listed until the agency learns of its closure, which may not occur until it seeks to arrange a biennial inspection.[1]

The Office of Applied Studies of the Substance Abuse and Mental Health Services Administration (SAMHSA), also conducts an annual (since 1992, biennial during 1987–1992) survey of methadone facilities called the National Drug and Alcoholism Treatment Unit Survey (NDATUS), data are reported by drug abuse and alcoholism treatment providers to their respective state agencies, which forward it to SAMHSA. The response rate has been between 80 and 85 percent. In this survey, methadone "units" are defined at state discretion. The term may refer to an individual facility or to a program consisting of a several separate facilities. This definition was adopted in 1987 to ease the states' reporting burden by allowing them to report data for an entire program, regardless of the number of clinical sites (or facilities), on a single survey form. The data on the number of patients in these units and the capacity and utilization of the units are unaffected by the manner in which units are counted.[2]

In 1992, NDATUS reported a total of 574 units (D. Melnick, SAMHSA, unpublished data, 1994). This was a decline in its unit count of nearly 10 percent over the period since 1987, from 633 to 574 units, which may be due to the reporting system. In 1992, FDA reported 737 active programs. FDA data show an increase in the number of active dispensing sites of 16 percent from

---

[1]FDA's count of inpatient detoxification programs is probably more accurate because most inpatient facilities have only one dispensing site. (E. Dory, FDA, personal communication, 1994)

[2]NDATUS has three other methodological limitations that need to be recognized (DHHS, 1993c). First, its data are more accurate for publicly funded facilities. State authorities are more likely to report information about units that receive state financing than about private units that receive no such funds. Second, some units do not respond for NDATUS is a voluntary survey. Third, NDATUS is not a complete listing of unit (Schmidt and Wiesner, 1993). Researchers who have sought to verify the listing through site visits to some cities have found that undercounting of up to 25 percent may have occurred (D'Aunno, University of Michigan, personal communication, 1994). With incomplete knowledge of the universe of U.S. providers, it is not known whether th units reporting to NDATUS are nationally representative. NDATUS is undergoing design improvements which over the next several years will yield greater accuracy and stronger linkages to states' client and financing data.

671 in 1987 to 737 in 1992 (E. Dory, FDA, personal communication, 1994). No reconciliation of these two counts has been attempted.

Regional Variation

The NDATUS data show strong regional variation in the distribution of methadone facilities and patients (based on the 1992 client census). Almost half of all U.S. methadone patients are found in the Northeast (46.6 percent); the West has 24.3 percent of all methadone patients; and the South and Midwest have the smallest percentages, with 16.1 percent and 13 percent, respectively (see Table 6-1). On a per capita basis, the Northeast has the highest rate of methadone patients at 94 per 100,000 population, followed by the West at 46, the Midwest at 22, and the South at 19 (see Table 6-1).

TABLE 6-1 Regional Distribution of Methadone Patients, 1992

Region	Number of Patients	Percentage of Total Patients	1992 Resident Population[a]	Patients per 1,000 Population[b]
West	25,124	24.3	55,108,000	0.46
Midwest	13,453	13	60,713,000	0.22
Northeast	48,230	46.6	51,118,000	0.94
South	16,687	16.1	88,143,000	0.19
Total	103,494[c]	100	255,082,000	0.41

[a]Bureau of the Census, 1993.
[b]This rate is based on the total regional resident population. A rate based on an opiate-addicted population might be different.
[c]This figure excludes Puerto Rico.

SOURCE: NDATUS, Office of Applied Studies, SAMHSA.

Underlying these regional differences are even greater differences by state. In 1992, California and New York, with 18,331[3] and 31,730 patient,[4] respectively, accounted for almost 50 percent of all methadone patients in the United States. Following these two, the states with the largest client censuses were Illinois, New Jersey, Massachusetts, Florida, Maryland, Michigan, and Texas. By contrast, the following 10 states did not report any methadone patients to NDATUS in 1992: Arkansas, Idaho, Maine, Mississippi, Montana, North Dakota, New Hampshire, South Dakota, Vermont, and West Virginia (D. Melnick, SAMHSA, unpublished data, 1994).

Number of Patients

In 1993, the most recent year for which national estimates of methadone patients were available, an estimated 117,000 patients received methadone treatment (Harwood et al., 1994). This figure is calculated from client counts reported to NDATUS in 1991, adjusted for the 82 percent response rate to the survey. A 1990 survey estimated the national total at 112,943 patients receiving methadone, of whom approximately 92 percent of patients were considered to be in maintenance and 8 percent in detoxification (Batten et al., 1993).

The total number of methadone patients has increased in the past five years, according to NDATUS. Between 1987 and 1992, the total number of patients grew by 27.6 percent (see Table 6-2). The client census was relatively stable between the mid1970s and the mid1980s, seesawing between 70,000 and 80,000 patients (IOM, 1990). The growth in patients since 1987 may be attributed to many factors—an increase in the survey response rate from 78 percent in 1987 to 85 percent in 1992, efforts to contain drug related crime, an expanded public health effort related to the AIDS and tuberculosis epidemics, and to a concern for drugrelated infant mortality. In addition, federal block grant expenditures for drug treatment grew during this period, accompanied by mandates to the states to ensure greater access to treatment (see below).

---

[3]This figure, reported to NDATUS in 1992, may include some outpatient methadone detoxification patients. California has a large outpatient detoxification population, as discussed below.

[4]These 31,730 clients represent data reported by 86 percent of the licensed methadone clinics. The 20(+) clinics that failed to complete a survey account for over 8,100 treatment slots.

Capacity and Utilization Rate

Paralleling an increasing number of patients was a reported increase of 47.6 percent in the average capacity (number of slots) of the methadone units reporting to NDATUS. The average number of methadone patients per unit (shown in Table 6-3) also increased by 40.8 percent. It is unclear whether these data mean that facilities are expanding to accommodate more patients, or that units are being consolidated administratively for reporting purposes, or both.

TABLE 6-2 Estimated Number of Methadone Patients by Facility Ownership, 1987–1992

Facility Ownership	1987	1989	1991	1992	% Rise 1987– 1992[a]
Private, for-profit	13,278	16,625	23,697	25,565	92.5
Private, not for-profit	51,096	56,338	54,969	60,428	18.2
State/local govt.	15,107	17,778	14,924	16,070	6.3
Federal govt.	2,371	1,493	1,696	2,440	2.9
Total	81,852	92,234	95,286	104,503	27.6

NOTE: Point prevalence estimates were taken on September 30, 1987, September 30, 1989, September 30, 1991, and September 30, 1992. Excluded are units that did not report methadone patients and capacity.

[a]These figures must be interpreted with some caution because of some small variation in the nonresponse rate from each year and because the number of private programs is incomplete.

SOURCE: NDATUS, Office of Applied Studies, SAMHSA.

NDATUS provides the only national data about methadone treatment capacity and utilization, important indicators of the availability of treatment.

Capacity, or the number of slots, is defined as the maximum number of active patients who could be enrolled. Utilization is calculated by dividing the number of actual patients by the capacity. These data must be interpreted cautiously, however, because NDATUS's definition of capacity[5] does not distinguish between a slot reserved for a private paying client and one for a publicly subsidized client. Private paying patients are believed to be underreported.

Nationwide, 122,442 methadone slots were reported to NDATUS in 1992, an increase from 1987, as can be seen in Table 6-4, paralleling the growth in the number of patients receiving methadone. Because the capacity and the number of patients have grown proportionally, methadone capacity utilization has remained steady at a high rate of 85–90 percent since 1987. Although a useful indicator, NDATUS's capacity utilization rate is not adjusted for differences in unit size. A special analysis of NDATUS's 1991 survey conducted by Lewin-VHI, Inc., yielded a weighted average utilization rate of 91.5 percent (based on 521 methadone treatment units that reported on both patients and capacity) (Lewin-VHI unpublished estimates, 1994).

TABLE 6-3 Size of Methadone Units, 1987–1992

	1987 (633 units)	1989 (729 Units)	1991 (527 units)	1992 (574 units)	% Increase 1987–1992[a]
Average capacity per unit	144.5	140.8	208.6	213.3	47.6
Average number of patients per unit	129.3	126.5	180.8	182.1	40.8

NOTE: Excludes units that did not report on methadone capacity.

[a]These percentage increases must be interpreted with some caution because the nonresponse rate varied slightly by year and because the number of private programs is incomplete.

SOURCE: NDATUS, Office of Applied Studies, SAMHSA.

---

[5]The instruction manual for NDATUS defines capacity as "the maximum number of individuals who could be enrolled as active clients . . . given the provider's staffing, funding, and physical facility at that time" (DHHS, 1991).

TABLE 6-4 Methadone Patients, Capacity, and Utilization, Nationwide, 1987–1992

	1987	1988	1991	1992
Patients receiving methadone	81,852	92,234	95,286	104,503
Methadone capacity[a]	91,495	102,646	109,906	122,442
Utilization rate[b]	89.5	89.9	86.7	85.3

[a]Capacity is the maximum number of individuals who could be enrolled as active patients on September 30 of the year of the survey. NDATUS's definition of capacity does not distinguish between slots reserved for private paying patients and publicly subsidized patients.
[b]Rate is number of methadone patients divided by reported capacity.

SOURCE: NDATUS, Office of Applied Studies, SAMHSA.

In California, the utilization rate varies according to whether the slot is reserved for private patients (who have private insurance or pay out-of-pocket) or for subsidized patients (those who receive mostly county, state, federal block grant, or Medicaid funding). California clinic operators identify their authorized slots according to the funding source: they reported in 1989 that 65 percent of the authorized slots were reserved for private patients and about 30 percent of slots were reserved for subsidized patients. The utilization rate (or occupancy rate) for the subsidized slots (95 percent) was higher than that for private slots (83 percent) (Goldstein, 1989), which has resulted in long waiting times for subsidized patients (see below). In New York, by contrast, no difference exists in the utilization rate for private and publicly financed slots, both being uniformly high at about 100 percent in 1994 (V. Fenlon, New York State Office of Alcoholism and Substance Abuse Services, unpublished data, 1994).

In 1992, the average methadone unit in the United States had an unweighted capacity of 213.3 slots and actually treated 182.1 patients, according to NDATUS (see Table 6-3), almost identical to the prior year. When the 1991 data were weighted to adjust for differences in unit size, a different picture emerges about each unit: the average client capacity was 337 slots and the average client census was 308 (Lewin-VHI unpublished estimates, 1994)[6]. The large difference between the nonweighted figures reported by NDATUS and those weighted by Lewin-VHI suggests that unit size is not uniformly distributed.

Waiting Lists

Although waiting times for admission to treatment programs led to the inclusion in the ADAMHA Reorganization Act of 1992 of a provision authorizing interim methadone maintenance treatment as a way to increase access to treatment, especially for intravenous drug users at risk of contracting AIDS (see discussion in chapter 5), the national data on waiting lists are not very good.[7]

Several national surveys on waiting lists suggest strong regional differences.[8] In New York City, for example, some facilities do have long waiting lists, which implies administrative or state regulatory limits on slots or program responses to limited financing.

A 1990 survey of client discharge records from drug treatment facilities, including 292 methadone facilities, based on a national sample drawn from NDATUS (Batten et al., 1992), found that 53.9 percent of methadone patients had no waiting time, 6.9 percent had a waiting time of less than seven days, and only 1.5 percent had waiting times of 14 or more days. However, the waiting time was not known or was not mentioned in 36.9 percent of client records. When facility ownership was examined, patients of private for-profit facilities were more likely to have no waiting time compared to those admitted to either private not-for-profit or publicly owned facilities (see Table 6-5).

---

[6]The Lewin-VHI analysis included 521 methadone treatment units from the 1991 NDATUS, which reported both clients and capacity, whereas the actual 1991 NDATUS averages were obtained from 527 programs, a very modest discrepancy that may explain some of the differences.

[7]This was acknowledged by FDA and NIDA in the 1989 proposed rule for interim methadone maintenance.

[8] Methodological problems include the possible difficulty of capturing addicts who may not place their names on a waiting list because of their belief that they will not gain admission. Survey information usually comes from clinic supervisors or client records—although neither source has information about prospective clients who wanted, but did not seek, admission. It is also difficult to know whether a client is wait-listed on more than one list at the same time.

TABLE 6-5 Waiting Time for Methadone Patients by Facility Type

	Publicly Owned (50 patients) N = 50	Private for Profit (63 patients) N = 63	Private Not for Profit (179 patients) N = 179	All Facilities (292 patients) N = 92
No waiting time	30.3%	89.2%	56.0%	53.9%
Waiting less than 7 days	3.5%	0.8%	11.7%	6.9%
Waiting 7–13 days	0.0%	0.0%	1.8%	0.9%
Waiting 14 or More Days	0.0%	0.0%	3.2%	1.5%
Unknown/not mentioned	66.3%	10.0%	27.3%	36.9%
Total	100%	100%	100%	100%

NOTE: Almost all percentages must be interpreted with caution because of a small sample size. Each percentage has been weighted to be nationally representative.

SOURCE: (Batten et al., 1992)

Waiting times were also addressed in a survey of 172 clinic directors conducted in 1990. The National Drug Abuse Treatment System Survey asked clinic directors to estimate the average waiting time for a client seeking admission to their clinic. Thirty-eight percent of clinics reported no waiting time; less than 7 days' average wait was estimated for 10 percent of the clinics; 7–14 days' average wait was estimated for 19 percent; and 15–95 days for 33 percent (T. D'Aunno, University of Michigan, unpublished data from the Drug Abuse Treatment System Survey). A substantial discrepancy exists between these figures and those in Table 6-5, suggesting the lack of uniform definitions and reporting methodologies.

The General Accounting Office (1990), in a small study of 24 methadone treatment programs, did not find a serious shortage of treatment slots.[9] Of the programs they evaluated, 14 did not have waiting lists and the other 10 programs had waits which ranged from one week to three months.

The GAO conclusion is amplified by data from New York and California. These states, which together account for almost 50 percent of U.S. methadone patients, maintain current registries of the number of patients on waiting lists, but not of waiting time. As of January 1994, New York State had 1,122 applicants on waiting lists for all methadone treatment programs, or 3 percent of the 40,292 patients in the state. About one-third of those were waiting for treatment at clinics operated by Beth Israel Hospital in New York City, whereas other facilities had waiting lists of fewer than 100 people (C.V. Fenlon, Office of Alcoholism and Substance Abuse Services, State of New York, unpublished data, 1994). However, New York State regards waiting lists as only one indication of demand for treatment.

California's monthly Drug Abuse Treatment Access Report, in March 1993, listed 2,488 applicants waiting for one of the 13,154 licensed methadone maintenance treatment slots (S. Nisenbaum, California Department of Alcohol and Drug Programs, unpublished data, 1994). Previously, a 1989 survey of all California clinic operators found that 58 percent of clinics kept a waiting list, and 1,077 applicants had waited an average of 6.6 to 7.1 months before entering treatment. Of these applicants, those entering private paying slots waited only 1.5 to 2 months, while those entering publicly funded slots waited 9 to 10 months (Goldstein, 1989). The situation appears to have improved. The state of California now estimates an average wait of 54 days for a subsidized treatment slot and notes that no waiting lists currently exist for private pay slots (S. Nisenbaum, 1994).

These data about waiting lists and times are not easy to interpret. Waiting lists vary regionally and between not-for-profit and for-profit facilities and no uniform definitions guide data collection. Although the data suggest a need for increased treatment capacity, they must be substantially improved in comprehensiveness and quality before they can provide much guidance for policy.

Facility Ownership

There are four general types of facility ownership (DHHS, 1993c): private for-profit facilities owned by an individual, partnership, or corporation; private

---

[9]The facilities in this small sample were selected because they were large, had operated for five years or more, and were in states with large intravenous drug populations.

not-for-profit facilities owned by a not-for-profit corporation, such as a church, a foundation, or another philanthropic group; state or local government facilities, typically owned by a county or city, although sometimes by a state government; and federal government facilities, most of which are administered by the Department of Veterans Affairs, the Federal prison system, or the U.S. Public Health Service.

NDATUS reports that most of the methadone units are owned by private, not-for-profit organizations. In 1992, there were almost three times as many private, not-for-profit units (321) as State/local units (107) and private, for-profit units (118) (D. Melnick, SAMHSA, unpublished data, 1994).

The share of treatment provided by different ownership types in terms of the number of patients treated is presented above in Table 6-2. The data shown in Table 6-2 yield percentages for 1992 as follows: about 58 percent of the patients were treated in private, not-for-profit units; about 24 percent in private, for-profit units; about 15 percent in state and local government units; and about 2 percent in federally operated units.

On the basis of client census data, the private, for-profit sector has more patients per unit per average than does the not-for-profit sector. This sector has also shown the largest growth of any ownership category in clients served. Table 6-2 shows a pronounced increase of 92.5 percent in the for-profit sector between 1987 and 1992, most of which has occurred in California, Texas, and Florida (see below). More modest growth has occurred in other ownership categories.

Four trends are apparent from this overview. First, the number of clients receiving methadone maintenance is increasing, especially those treated in private, for-profit facilities. Second, the growth in the client population has been accompanied by a growth in treatment capacity, mostly by increases in the size of existing facilities. Third, facility utilization remains high, especially in publicly supported facilities. Fourth, few new programs have been established (owing often to restrictive zoning regulations and community opposition).

FINANCING OF METHADONE TREATMENT

Methadone treatment is financed from a combination of federal, state, and private sources, and the combination varies markedly by state and by program. On the national level, NDATUS collects expenditure data on methadone treatment that are separate from overall alcohol and drug treatment data. Although available on data tapes, these data are not otherwise easily accessible to the public.

Estimates of expenditures for methadone treatment for fiscal year 1993 have recently been made by Harwood and his colleagues at Lewin-VHI (Harwood et al., 1994), using 1991 NDATUS financial information adjusted for inflation. The annual payments from all sources for methadone maintenance treatment is estimated by Harwood et al. at $480 million in FY 1993. This estimate, which does not include inpatient detoxification, assumes that 117,000 patients are receiving outpatient treatment at an average annual treatment cost of $4,100 per patient. Of this amount, the cost of the medication represents a very small fraction, about $4–8 per client per week (P. Coulis, National Institute of Drug Abuse, personal communication, 1994), or about 7 percent of treatment costs. The bulk of treatment costs are for counseling services and other administrative, recordkeeping, and regulatory costs. The introduction of LAAM is expected to double the per patient cost of the medication (G. DeVaux, BioDevelopment Corp., personal communication, 1994).

The Lewin-VHI unpublished estimates fiscal year for methadone mainte-nance for fiscal year 1993 divide the $480 million total cost into three major components (see Figure 6-1). First, public funding accounts for $386 million, or 80 percent of the total, consisting of federal block grant funds, state alcohol and substance abuse funds, Medicaid and local funds. Second, out-of-pocket payments by patients account for $82 million, or 17 percent of the total. Third, private insurance pays for $12 million, or 2.5 percent of the total.

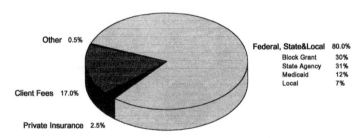

FIGURE 6-1 Payments for methadone treatment, 1993. Total payments = $480 million. Adapted from 1991 NDATUS by Lewin-VHI. SOURCES: Butynski et al (1994); Harwood et al. (1994); and DHHS (1993).

Public financing of *all* substance abuse treatment (for alcohol and drug abuse), which accounts for 80 percent of all financing, includes three components—state agency funding, federal block grants, and Medicaid, all of which are administered by state agencies. Financing from all sources of all state alcohol and drug abuse programs that receive some state funding is surveyed annually in the State Alcohol and Drug Abuse Profile (SADAP), administered since 1987 by the National Association of State Alcohol and Drug Abuse Directors, Inc. (NASADAD). The survey does not include all programs; it has virtually no data on private for-profit programs, some not-for-profit programs, and Department of Veterans Affairs programs (DHHS, 1993d). Also, data are not disaggregated by treatment modality, such as methadone maintenance. The SADAP survey shows that public financing in fiscal year 1991 accounted for about 78 percent of alcohol and drug abuse expenditures for treatment programs receiving some state support (see data in Table 6-6).

TABLE 6-6 Trends in Financing of State-Supported Alcohol and Other Drug Abuse Services by Largest Funding Sources

Year	Federal Block Grant	State Alcohol/ Drug Agency	Private Insurance Client Fees[a]	Medicaid and Other Public Sources[b]
1987	15%	45%	22%	9%
1988	17%	43%	20%	11%
1989	20%	42%	18%	12%
1990	22.2%	37.8%	15.7%	16.6%
1991	29.2%	34.7%	15.5%	13.7%
1992	30.2%	32.8%	18.1%	12.3%

NOTE: Data are from the State Alcohol and Drug Abuse Profile (SADAP), administered by the National Association of State Alcohol and Drug Abuse Director, Inc.

Also includes court fines. This column includes the same information as the SADAP category called "Other Sources."

This column combines the SADAP categories, "Other State Agency" and "Other Federal Government," in order to capture the federal and state shares of Medicaid, which constitute most of these two categories. There are other state and federal funds included in this column, but they do not come from the Federal block grant or from state substance abuse agencies.

SOURCE: DHHS, 1993d.

TABLE 6-7 Federal Block Grant and State Alcohol/Drug Agency Expenditures Reported for State-Supported Alcohol and Other Drug Abuse Services

Year	Federal Block Grant	State Alcohol/ Drug Agency
1987	$272,570,630	$819,807,824
1988	$355,025,431	$910,134,922
1989	$474,677,106	$1,009,099,083
1990	$645,477,081	$1,099,253,225
1991	$946,468,801	$1,126,634,230

SOURCE: DHHS, 1993d.

State agency funding, since 1987, has been the largest single component of all state substance abuse expenditures. In 1992, funds from state alcohol and drug agencies accounted for 32.8 percent of all alcohol and drug abuse services according to SADAP (Table 6-6). Valued at about $1.1 billion in 1991 (Table 6-7), this represents the largest single financing component. The state share actually declined from 1987 (45 percent) to 1992 as federal block grants increased more rapidly (Table 6-6).

Federal block grant funding has assumed an increasingly prominent role in the overall financing of substance abuse services. Table 6-6 shows that in 1992 block grants accounted for 30.2 percent of all substance abuse funding, up from 1987, when it accounted for 15 percent of the total. Between 1987 and 1991, state agencies reported an increase in block grant revenues from about $273 million to nearly $1 billion (Table 6-7).[10] Since the establishment

---

[10]Alcohol Drug Abuse and Mental Health (ADM) block grants were authorized by the Omnibus Budget Reconciliation Act of 1981, which reflected the Reagan administration's decision to give states greater control in the provision of mental health and substance abuse services. The ADM block grant is a "no strings attached" grant to each state. It reversed federal government policies of the 1970s, through which categorical grants gave the federal government a central role in all aspects of alcoholism, substance abuse, and mental health services. A historical description of the

of the block grant in 1981, federal legislation has changed its underlying philosophy toward a stronger federal role in monitoring how funds are spent and in holding states accountable. [11] The federal block grant requires that states give priority to intravenous drugs users, persons of color, ethnic minorities, women, especially women with children.

Medicaid is an important source of funding for methadone treatment, but one that is extremely difficult to measure (IOM, 1990; Solloway, 1992; Horgan et al, forthcoming). States have great discretion in determining substance abuse coverage and they are not required to report substance abuse expenditures, let alone those for methadone, to the Health Care Financing Administration, which oversees Medicaid.

Nevertheless, estimates are available concerning Medicaid's contribution to treatment. According to SADAP, federal and state Medicaid accounts for, at most, 12.3 percent of *all* alcohol and drug abuse funding (Table 6-6). An estimate of Medicaid financing specifically for methadone treatment has been made by the Drug Services Research Survey (DSRS) of Brandeis University. This two-phase survey of a national sample of drug treatment facilities (phase I) and client discharge records (phase II) revealed that about 8 percent of total revenues for all drug treatments were from Medicaid (Horgan et al., 1994). When methadone client records were examined, Medicaid was listed as the expected source of payment for 27 percent[12] of these patients upon admission (Batten et al., 1992). Medicaid-certified methadone facilities received about 30 percent of their revenues from Medicaid, a percentage greater than nonmethadone treatment facilities that were also Medicaid-certified (Horgan et al., 1994).

Department of Veterans Affairs

The Department of Veterans Affairs (VA) sponsors one of the world's largest networks of hospitals and outpatient clinics. There are an estimated 27 million beneficiaries served at 171 hospitals and 220 outpatient facilities nationwide. Although all veterans and their dependents are eligible for care, the highest priority is accorded to those veterans whose illnesses or injuries are a direct result of military service (i.e., "service-connected veterans") or low-income veterans who are not "service-connected." Substance abusers are most

---

respective funding roles of federal and state governments is found in *Treating Drug Problems* (IOM, 1990).

[11]See the Anti-Drug Abuse Acts of 1986 and 1988 and the ADAMHA Reorganization Act of 1992.

[12]The figure of 27 percent represents a weighted percentage so as to be nationally representative, but it must be interpreted with caution because of the small sample size.

likely to become eligible via the low-income requirement, rather than the service-connected requirement. The VA is obligated to provide hospital and some outpatient care to high priority veterans, and, if space is available, they may provide care to other eligible veterans who do not qualify as high priority. In practice, only a small percentage of lower priority veterans receive care.

In the wake of criticism that the VA has insufficient capacity to treat veterans with substance abuse disorders (IOM, 1990), Congress gave the VA additional appropriations in fiscal year 1990 to expand and enhance treatment capacity. Patients diagnosed with alcohol or drug abuse represent one of the most frequently discharged groups of patients from VA medical centers (VAMCs), second only to those with heart disease (Department of Veterans Affairs, 1991). A total of 26 percent of all VA inpatients were diagnosed with a primary or secondary substance abuse disorder (Peterson et al., 1993). Although much is known about the characteristics and costs of the inpatient substance abuse population, the VA did not collect data until recently about the number of outpatient substance abuse patients, including methadone patients, and their cost of care.

In 1993, the first year for which data were available, a total of 5,886 patients nationwide received methadone maintenance treatment at approximately 36 VAMCs (R. Swindle, Program Evaluation Resource Center, Palo Alto VAMC, personal communication, 1994). These patients are approximately 5 percent of all U.S. methadone patients. Trend data are unavailable. Most VA methadone patients are low-income veterans whose opiate dependence is not service-connected, but who may have another ailment that is service-connected.

The VA estimates that the overall cost of outpatient methadone maintenance treatment was about $22 million in fiscal year 1993 (Department of Veterans Affairs, 1993). This estimate is based on an average outpatient visit cost of $36.65 for all types of substance abuse treatment; the average cost of an outpatient methadone visit, though not determined, it is likely to be lower (R. Swindle, Program Evaluation Resource Center, Palo Alto VAMC, personal communication, 1994). There were over 607,000 outpatient methadone visits in 1993.

The VA plays an important role in research on treatments for drug abuse. Through an interagency agreement with the National Institute on Drug Abuse, the VA sponsors large-scale clinical trials for new medications. For example, the VA was a major participant in the clinical trial that led to the approval of LAAM for opiate addiction.

Out-of-Pocket and Private Insurance

Private funding of methadone treatment consists of patient out-of-pocket expenditures and private insurance through a third party carrier or a prepaid plan. Based on 1991 NDATUS data, Harwood estimates that out-of-pocket expenditures constitute 17 percent of the total, private insurance 2.5 percent (Harwood et al., 1994). All private sources make up nearly onefifth of methadone treatment expenditures (see Figure 6-1). This percentage is quite similar to the SADAP estimate for all reported substance abuse expenditures.

Patient out-of-pocket payments are a source of treatment financing, although data are not readily available. The DSRS survey, phase II, of client records for all types of drug treatment facilities (described earlier) analyzed the expected source of client payments at the time of admission. Although the sample of methadone patients was small, the findings in Table 6-8 show that 30.8 percent of methadone patients in all facilities were expected to pay for treatment out-of-pocket ("self-pay"). The DSRS survey included a sample of private for-profit facilities. When the methadone client data were stratified by facility type, it was found that 77.2 percent of patients in private for-profit facilities were expected to pay out-of-pocket (Table 6-8), a far greater percentage than patients at other types of methadone facilities.

Data reported by a sample of clinic directors in a 1990 survey reflect differences between for-profit and not-for-profit clinics with respect to client out-of-pocket payment. Fiftyseven percent of private for-profit clinics derive 80 percent or more of their revenues from client out-of-pocket payments. In contrast, 73 percent of private not-for-profit clinics obtain 20 percent or less of their revenues from client payments (T. D'Aunno, unpublished data from the Drug Abuse Treatment System Survey). Similarly, based on an analysis of NDATUS, the IOM (1990) found that 75 percent of revenues at private for-profit facilities were from client out-of-pocket payments.

Private insurance appears to represent a very small component of client financing. The DSRS survey found that 4.4 percent of methadone patients at all facilities were expected at admission to be covered by private health insurance and an additional 1.9 percent by an HMO or other prepaid plan (Table 6-8). In comparison to patients receiving other types of drug treatment, methadone patients were the least likely to have private health insurance coverage. For example, approximately 30 percent of patients in hospital inpatient drug abuse programs were expected to be covered by private health insurance (Batten et al, 1992).

TABLE 6-8   Percentage Distribution of Methadone Patients by Primary Source of Payment and Facility Type

	Publicly Owned (50 pts.)	Private for-profit (63 pts.)	Private not for-profit (179 pts.)	All Facilities (292 pts.)
Public subsidy	2.6%	0.0%	7.1%	4.2%
Philanthropy	0.0%	0.0%	0.0%	0.0%
No payment, un-specified	0.0%	0.0%	0.4%	0.2%
Self-pay	11.5%	77.2%	25.5%	30.8%
HMO/other pre-paid plan	0.0%	3.6%	2.6%	1.9%
Private health insurance	1.3%	0.0%	8.3%	4.4%
Medicaid	29.1%	15.6%	30.2%	27.0%
Medicare	3.5%	0.0%	1.2%	1.7%
Other federal (DOD, Champus, VA)	2.9%	0.0%	1.2%	1.5%
Social services	1.3%	2.8%	0.9%	1.4%
Other	1.3%	0.0%	16.9%	8.5%
Not permitted to abstract	0.0%	0.0%	0.0%	0.0%
Unknown/not mentioned	46.7%	0.9%	5.8%	18.4%

NOTE: Almost all percentages must be interpreted with caution because of a small sample size.
SOURCE: Batten et al., 1992.

*   *   *   *   *

The previous two sections have examined the characteristics and the financing of the methadone treatment system. The system has been growing over the last several years, in contrast to relative stability from the mid-1970s to the mid-1980s. Increases occurred in the number of patients, the number of slots, and the number of facilities. The growth is most pronounced in the for-profit sector, which nearly doubled the number of patients between 1987 and 1992. The utilization rate remains exceedingly high, giving rise to waiting lists at many clinics, particularly those that receive large public subsidies. The time spent on a waiting list, which is difficult to evaluate on a nationwide basis, has exceeded several months in some studies. Data about facility utilization, waiting time, and the demand for treatment is needed for policymakers, but good national data on these matters do not currently exist.

Most of the estimated $480 million in total treatment expenditures comes from public sources, such as state substance abuse agencies, federal block grants, and Medicaid. Private out-of-pocket payments account for an estimated 17 percent of the total, and private insurance accounts for the smallest portion, only 2.5 percent of the total (Lewin-VHI, unpublished estimates, 1994).

STATE SUBSTANCE ABUSE AGENCIES[13]

An important role in the overall substance abuse treatment system, including methadone treatment, is played by state governments. The states are engaged in the regulation and financing of methadone treatment; the licensing of practitioners; quality assurance; data collection; and various activities related to the control of illicit drugs, the general use of controlled substances, and the control of the diversion of methadone.

State government substance abuse activities are quite variable. Although states must adhere to the federal methadone regulations, they may also mandate additional, more restrictive, measures. Some of the most common measures adopted by states concern admission criteria, staffing ratios, take-home policies, dosing limits, treatment duration, and patient rights. Not surprisingly, the patterns vary substantially from state to state.

Variation across the states is also apparent in how treatment is financed. States can and do exercise much latitude in public financing of methadone treatment, using an array of federal, state, and local funds, as discussed in the

---

[13]Much of the material in this section is based on an analysis of state regulations and on interviews conducted in January 1994 with key state administrators, who are listed at the end of this chapter.

previous section. The states are not permitted to use federal block grant funds to finance treatment at private, for-profit clinics, however, nor are they usually permitted to use their own state agency funds for this purpose. (These clinics receive most of their revenues from client fees and Medicaid.)

In addition to variability, there is a notable absence of systematic data on state substance abuse programs. Therefore, in this section, we examine how methadone is regulated and financed by five states with large methadone client populations: New York, California, Illinois, Florida, and Massachusetts. (Data for these five states for the period 1987–1992 are shown in Table 6-9.) How these States will regulate and finance LAAM, a newly approved treatment for opiate addiction, is not yet known, as these states have yet to take all of the necessary regulatory steps towards its introduction.

New York

As of October 1994, the state of New York had over 40,000 methadone maintenance patients, the largest patient population in the U.S., and double that of California, the next largest. In New York this patient population is treated in 148 methadone treatment facilities, of which 114 are voluntary (private) not-for-profit clinics and 34 are for-profit clinics. (There are no state-owned or -operated clinics.) One not-for-profit clinic specializes in the treatment of pregnant addicts and another one in the treatment of adolescent addicts. All clinics are licensed and regulated by the New York State Office of Alcoholism and Substance Abuse Services (OASAS). Apparently because of community opposition, only 3 new methadone clinics have been licensed in New York State in the past 20 years (personal communication, Marguerite Saunders, Commissioner, Office of Alcoholism and Substance Abuse Services).

In January 1994, the not-for-profit clinics had a patient census of 30,662 and the for-profits, 9,265 (V. Fenlon, New York State Office of Alcoholism and Substance Abuse Services, unpublished data, 1994.) The average clinic census is 269 patients; in New York City, five clinics have a license capacity greater than 550.

Financing

New York State compiles financing information for voluntary, not-for profit clinics, for which total expenditures in 1992–1993 were about $139. million (see Table 6-10).

TABLE 6-9 Patients Receiving Methadone, Methadone Capacity, and Capacity Utilization Rate in Five States

	Patients Receiving Methadone				Methadone Capacity[a]				Utilization Rate[b]			
	1987	1989	1991	1992	1987	1989	1991	1992	1987	1989	1991	1992
California	12,052	12,828	18,352	18,331	14,139	15,129	22,426	23,812	85.2	84.8	81.8	77.0
Florida	1,445	1,770	2,767	2,712	1,734	2,199	3,746	4,141	83.3	80.5	73.9	65.5
Illinois	3,170	3,250	4,717	4,775	3,945	3,657	5,452	5,436	80.4	88.9	86.5	87.8
Massachusetts	390	1,389	3,576	3,814	502	1,876	4,144	4,397	77.7	74.0	86.3	86.7
New York[c]	34,374	33,363	29,159	31,730	34,059	34,003	30,595	33,520	100.9	98.1	95.3	94.7

[a]Capacity is the maximum number of individuals who could be enrolled as active patients on September 30 of each year when the survey was conducted.

[b]Methadone capacity utilization rate is obtained by dividing the number of methadone patients by the capacity.

[c]These figures underestimate the total by approximately 20 percent, according to the associate commissioner for health and planning of the New York State Office of Alcoholism and Substance Abuse Services. For example, the 1992 figure is estimated at 40,000 patients receiving methadone.

SOURCE: NDATUS, Office of Applied Studies, SAMHSA.

TABLE 6-10 Financing of Methadone Treatment in Publicly
Funded Clinics in New York State, Fiscal Year 1992–1993

Revenue Source	Amount	Percent of Total
OASAS state aid[a]	$ 20,441,600	14.6
Federal block grant	$ 20,964,500	15.0
Medicaid	$ 87,142,500	62.4
Patient fees	$ 3,630,900	2.6
Local tax	$ 2,940,800	2.1
All other	$ 4,427,400	3.3
Total Financing	$139,547,700	100

NOTE: Publicly funded clinics are private not-for-profit clinics.
Data on private insurance revenues are not included, but are considered
to be negligible by state administrators.

[a]Office of Alcoholism and Substance Abuse Services.

SOURCE: Addie Corradi, Associate Commissioner, Health and Planning
Services Division, New York State OASAS.

Medicaid accounts for 62.4 percent of this total, far higher than the
national average of 12 percent, followed by the federal block grant at 15
percent and the OASAS state aid at 14.6 percent. Patient fees accounted for an
estimated 2.6 percent of treatment costs. Although data were not available or
private insurance, it is considered negligible by state administrators. The
average cost of treatment in New York State is estimated at $4,500 per client
per year.

New York has liberal eligibility requirements for Medicaid and financing
comes from federal, state, and local governments. Consequently, Medicaid
expenditures for methadone maintenance are not evenly divided between the
state and the federal government. In fact, state and local funds constitute 8(
percent of all Medicaid expenditures because many patients are not eligible for
federal matching funds but are eligible under more generous state criteria

Patients in treatment programs are generally eligible for federal Medicaid
dollars when they qualify for aid for dependent children (AFDC), supplemental
security income (SSI), and Medically Needy programs. Yet, because of stric

categorical and income criteria, many patients are ineligible for these programs.

In New York, however, patients may also obtain Medicaid coverage by qualifying for Home Relief, which provides state-only Medicaid funds. Sixty percent of Medicaid-enrolled methadone patients in New York State receive Home Relief, which also provides cash assistance for low-income people and is designed to maintain them in the community.

Recognizing that the New York share of total Medicaid expenditures is unusually high, state administrators are seeking through a pilot program to shift their costs to federal Medicaid. The pilot program helps disabled patients receiving Home Relief to qualify for SSI and thereby become eligible for federal Medicaid.

All voluntary, not-for-profit clinics qualify for state agency funds, for whom the state is the "payer of last resort." Once Medicaid, client fees, and private insurance have been obtained, the remaining costs at these publicly funded clinics are covered by state Office of Alcoholism and Substance Abuse Services funds and federal block grant funds so they do not operate at a deficit.

Regulations

New York State methadone regulations are similar to the federal regulations, but diverge in four important areas: staffing ratios, urine testing, client rights, and central registries. The state also provides certain additional services: since 30 percent of patient admissions to methadone clinics are HIV positive, and thus at high risk for tuberculosis, New York sponsors active methadone clinic-based programs for the onsite delivery of tuberculosis medication.

With respect to staffing, one full-time doctor is required for every 300 patients. Two full-time nurses are required for the first 300 patients, but thereafter another full-time nurse is required for each additional 100 patients or fraction thereof. One full-time case worker is required to counsel every 50 patients.

Urine testing is required on a weekly basis for the first three months in treatment. If the testing reveals no indication of drug abuse, patients may be placed on a monthly urine testing schedule. In contrast, the Federal regulations require eight random urine tests during the first year of treatment.

Patients have protections against involuntary termination from treatment. Patients must be informed in writing of the reasons for their discharge and of their right to request a review of the termination decision. They may appeal the decision before the program is allowed to begin the discharge process, according to OASAS regulations. This discharge process typically involves detoxification treatment with decreasing doses of methadone. During detoxification, the dosage may not be lowered more than 10 mg every three days.

Finally, the regulations mandate a central registry system, which is designed to prevent enrollment of a patient in more than one methadone program. Before an applicant can enroll in a program, the program is required to submit information to the central registry. The registry also maintains uptodate information about patient discharges and transfers.

California

In California, all state financing, regulatory, and licensing functions related to alcohol and substance abuse are carried out by the Department of Alcohol and Drug Programs. The state of California has the second largest methadone client population in the United States. In 1994, about 20,000 methadone maintenance patients were treated at any one time, including those in temporary treatment slots authorized by the state to respond to the AIDS epidemic. The number of patients receiving methadone grew substantially between 1987 and 1992, increasing by 52 percent (see Table 6-9).

The treatment population size is much smaller than the estimated opiate addict population. Earlier research estimates were that California enrolled fewer than 8 percent of its opiate addicts in treatment (Anglin and McGlothlin 1985; Goldstein, 1991). More recently, the state of California estimates that approximately 15 percent of opiate addicts are in the treated population (S. Nisenbaum, State of California, unpublished data, 1992).

As of November 1994, the state of California licensed 117 facilities to dispense methadone. Within these facilities are 222 licensed programs, each facility usually having more than one program (defined under FDA regulations as a dispensing site). Among the 222 programs, 117 are outpatient methadone maintenance, 104 are outpatient detoxification, and one is an inpatient detoxification program.

The large proportion of *outpatient* detoxification programs is unique because in many other states detoxification is usually provided on an inpatient basis or at the end of maintenance treatment. California regulations and financing have encouraged outpatient detoxification programs, in which patients receive tapered methadone doses to bring them to a drug-free state within 21 days, while also undergoing periodic medical evaluation and counseling. Between July 1, 1992, and June 30, 1993, a total of 63,832 episodes of methadone detoxification were provided in approximately 5,500 state-licensed slots (J. Jarfors, State of California, unpublished data, 1994).

State officials are exploring the feasibility of revising its 21-day detoxification regulation to conform to federal regulations that permit long-term detoxification up to 180 days.

California providers include many private, for-profit facilities and programs. Of the 117 methadone facilities in the state, over half are private, not-for-profit (57 percent), but almost a third are private, for-profit (31 percent). A small proportion, 12 percent, are publicly operated by counties; the state does not own or operate any facilities. According to state officials, most new programs are private, not-for-profit.

Financing

While the Department of Alcohol and Drug Programs maintains information on the public funding allocated to methadone programs, a considerable portion of overall expenditures for methadone treatment is not included in the department's figures because as many as 75 percent of treatment slots are fee-for-service, payments for which are not required to be reported to the state. Licensed clinics do report their monthly slot fees in their annual renewal applications. In July 1993, these averaged about $200 a month for methadone maintenance and $248 per 21-day detoxification episode.

Public funding for drug treatment in California has traditionally come from state general funds, federal block grants, and Drug MediCal. The former two sources of funds are combined into a funding stream known as Drug Allocation Money, which is allocated among California counties according to a complex formula and requires a 10 percent match from county revenues. Counties may spend their drug allocation on drug treatment and prevention in any way they choose, provided that they meet any categorical funding stipulations attached to such funds. Thus, counties determine which types of treatment they will provide under their drug allocation money; a number of counties have chosen not to fund methadone programs. Even in counties that do fund methadone treatment, subsidized slots have in recent years largely been limited to patients who are HIV-positive, pregnant women, and other specified categories.

The other major source of public funding for methadone treatment has been Drug MediCal, a program that counties may "opt into" in order to provide drug treatment for individuals who are eligible for MediCal. Drug MediCal differs from regular MediCal. Under regular MediCal, the state matches federal Medicaid dollar for dollar to pay for the medical care of eligible individuals. Under Drug MediCal, before July 1, 1994, the state provided counties with federal Medicaid allocations, which the counties were required to match dollar for dollar from their state-generated allocations. As an incentive to the counties to "opt into" Drug MediCal, the state does not require 10 percent matching on the portion of a county's State Drug Allocation Money that the county uses to match Federal Medicaid funds. Again, the counties have decided which types of treatment will be funded under Drug MediCal.

In 1994, Drug MediCal policies were undergoing change owing to a lawsuit in which the court ruled that persons who qualify for MediCal are entitled to receive methadone maintenance if they otherwise meet eligibility requirements for admission, and a certified program had available capacity. While the details of this new financing system are still being worked out, currently state general funds are being made available to the counties to pay for the treatment of MediCal recipients, including those who qualify for methadone treatment; any funds left over can be used to fund treatment slots for other people in need of treatment who are not MediCal eligible. The full impact of this change will not be known for several years, but it promises to be far-reaching.

Regulations

The state of California has numerous treatment regulations, in effect since 1973, which cover admission criteria, the authorized number of treatment slots, take-home policies, detoxification treatment, staffing, treatment planning, multiple registration, urinalysis, maximum dosage levels, and duration of treatment, all of which are described below.

In order to be admitted into a program, prospective patients must be currently addicted and have a two-year addiction history. This two-year history requirement contrasts with the federal and New York requirement of a one-year history. Potential patients must also have evidence of two prior failures in withdrawal treatment with regimens other than methadone maintenance (California Code of Regulations, Title 9). In response to concerns about HIV transmission, however, California regulations now permit waiver of state admission criteria and allow the use of federal criteria, on a program-by-program basis.

Under the same regulations, the state limits the number of permanent and temporary slots for methadone maintenance and detoxification. A facility can only be licensed for up to 150 permanent detoxification and 300 permanent maintenance slots, and may exceed licensed capacity by 10 percent for emergency admissions. In January 1994, the state licensed 17,639 permanent maintenance and 2,455 temporary maintenance slots. With respect to methadone detoxification, the state licensed 5,337 permanent and 52 temporary slots.

California regulations permit temporary increases in capacity on a program-by-program basis. The licensure of temporary slots and/or the waiver of state admission criteria are recent regulatory responses designed to expand access to treatment primarily because of the HIV and AIDS epidemic. The only difference between a permanent and temporary slot is that the latter has provision for HIV counseling. Patients in temporary slots benefit from the same staffing ratio and counseling requirements as those in permanent slots. (Temporary slots licensed by the state are not the same as slots for "interim methadone maintenance," which were authorized under the ADAMHA Reorganization Act of 1992 in FDA regulations of January 1993.)

California's regulations are more stringent than federal regulations regarding take-home policies. After the first three months of treatment, federal regulations allow a maximum two-day take-home supply of methadone; California, by comparison, allows a one-day supply. The maximum takehome supply under federal regulations is for six days, if the client has satisfactorily adhered to treatment rules for three consecutive years. In contrast, the California maximum is three days, reached only after two years of treatment.

In terms of staffing, the state requires one physician for every 200 patients and one counselor for every 40 patients. There are no specific licensure requirements for counselors, but they are required to receive ongoing training. Programs are required to review patient treatment plans every 90 days "with the objective of reducing the dosage level." Under federal regulations, treatment plans are required to be reviewed every 90 days during the first year; thereafter, only a twice-a-year review is needed.

To prevent multiple enrollments, and thus limit the possibility of methadone diversion, California mandates a two-tiered process: (1) Upon admission, urinalysis is conducted to identify whether methadone, or its metabolite, are present. If the results are positive, program administrators must contact other methadone programs within a 50-mile radius. (2) Each client is assigned a number that is checked against a statewide data base to ensure that he or she has only enrolled once.

Once admitted to treatment, patients are required to undergo urinalysis every 30 days, a frequency greater than the federal requirement of at least eight times a year. By statute, providers are not permitted under any circumstances to exceed a daily methadone dose of 180 mg. Although the state imposes a two-year limit on maintenance treatment unless a physician certifies that continued treatment is medically justified, almost all patients who reach this limit are evaluated and, on the basis of a determination by the physician, continue treatment beyond two years. If patients are involuntarily discharged from a program, state regulations ensure a fair hearing.

Florida

In Florida, the state Alcohol, Drug Abuse, and Mental Health Office is responsible for technical assistance, oversight, and policy formulation pertaining to methadone treatment at its central office, but all licensing and distribution of public funds are handled by 15 state district offices. There are approximately 2,700 methadone patients in Florida, according to the 1992 NDATUS (see Table 6-9).

A total of 22 methadone clinics operate in Florida, one of which is publicly owned; the remainder are privately owned. Sixteen of the latter are private, for-profit, and five are not for-profit. For-profit facilities have increased from six in 1986 to 16 in 1994.

Financing

State funds and federal block grant funds finance only not-for-profit clinics, and no for-profit ones. Of the $1.9 million in revenues received by not-for-profit clinics from July 1, 1992, through June 30, 1993, client fees and insurance accounted for 36 percent, one-fifth (19.9 percent) was from state agency and block grant funds, 17.7 percent from local matching funds, and 12.7 percent from Medicaid.[14] Medicaid pays for all methadone services, including a dispensing fee, but not for the prescription itself.

Some private, for-profit clinics accept only client fees as payment for services; they do not accept private insurance or Medicaid, and they are ineligible to receive state agency and block grant funding.

The average annual cost of treatment in Florida in private, not-for-profit units ranges from about $2,600 to 3,200. Private for-profit providers charge approximately $9.00 a day, but the state does not compile funding figures for these clinics since they receive no state funds.

Regulations

Florida regulates certain aspects of methadone treatment more stringently than the federal regulations. Within the next several months, however, the state plans a complete revision of these regulations. Current regulations require one staff member for every 45 patients and restrictive takehome policies. Florida also requires a central registry and strict quality assurance. Finally, current

---

[14]State reports do not specify whether the local matching funds were designated for block grant or Medicaid funding.

regulations prohibit clinics from turning away applicants who meet federal admission criteria; if space is unavailable, they are placed on a waiting list.

Illinois

In 1994, approximately 6,000 patients received methadone maintenance treatment in Illinois (see Table 6-9). Illinois has 36 methadone programs, of which 28 are private, not-for-profit and eight are private, for-profit. In the past several years, 80 percent of newly licensed programs have been for-profit. Most clinics in Illinois have waiting lists for patients wishing to enter treatment. Waiting times vary from a few day to several months. All licensing, monitoring, and program coordination are orchestrated by the Illinois Department of Alcoholism and Substance Abuse.

Financing

The 29 private, not-for-profit clinics received $10.7 million from state agency and block grant funds and $6.03 million from Medicaid in fiscal 1993, but state administrators had no information on client fees and private insurance. Medicaid funding in Illinois has expanded over the past 3–4 years, initially covering only medication and counseling costs and now covering dispensing fees, medical examinations, and urine testing. In the future, state officials expect the Medicaid program to impose limits on the amount of methadone services it covers during a one-year period. Private, for-profit clinics are not permitted to receive state agency and block grant funding. The average client cost in not-for-profit facilities in Illinois ranges from $2,500 to 3,000 per year.

Regulations

Illinois has extensive state regulations for all alcoholism and substance abuse programs, with which methadone clinics must comply. These regulations cover such areas as client rights, quality assurance, and research. For example, each program must have a written statement that describes patient rights, including the route of appeal available when a client objects to a facility's decisions, policies, or procedures.

Illinois methadone regulations require programs to comply with the federal methadone regulations and add only one additional requirement: a client is not allowed to receive more than a 3-day take-home supply of medication without a written exemption from the Department of Alcoholism and Substance Abuse.

Massachusetts

In 1992, there were about 3,800 methadone patients in the state of Massachusetts (see Table 6-9). In the state, 14 agencies operate a total of 29 licensed methadone facilities, including 21 sites, 2 satellites, and 7 medication units. These agencies hold 12 outpatient and two inpatient licenses. Neither the state nor the counties own methadone facilities. Private, for-profit clinics are eligible to receive state funds.

The Massachusetts Bureau of Substance Abuse Services licenses each methadone facility to administer methadone. Separate licensing is required to provide counseling at these facilities, as is true for all substance abuse and mental health treatment centers in the state.

Financing

Providers are paid by the Bureau of Substance Abuse Services and Medicaid at a rate of $9.61 per day per patient for medical assessment, drug dispensing, and case management. Individual counseling is reimbursed at a rate of $51 for a 60-minute session; group counseling is reimbursed at $20 per person for a 90-minute session.

Massachusetts permits the use of its substance abuse funds, but not its block grant funds, to finance treatment at private, for-profit facilities. Although the number of for-profit facilities is small, this is a significant departure from many other states. The average cost of treatment in Massachusetts is $5,000 per year or $2,500 for a 180-day episode.

Medicaid contributes a large percentage (53 percent) of the $13 million in revenues that methadone providers reported to the state. This reliance on Medicaid is similar to that of New York State, in which Medicaid contributes 60 percent of treatment costs at publicly funded clinics, but unlike most states, for which Medicaid accounts for only 12 percent of treatment costs. Massachusetts Medicaid expenditures are evenly matched between federal and state sources. The Bureau of Substance Abuse Services contributes $5 million or 38.5 percent of the total, of which 75 percent comes from legislative appropriations and 25 percent from federal block grant funds. Client fees account for $0.8 million or 6 percent of the total, and private insurance for

$0.3 million or 2.3 percent of the total. The Bureau is the "payer of last resort," as is New York State.

Regulations

Methadone providers in Massachusetts must adhere to treatment requirements under both the Massachusetts Code of Regulations and the contract performance standards that were established as conditions of Medicaid and Bureau funding. State regulations require clinics to be open seven days a week and two hours outside of normal working hours. They also require more frequent treatment reviews than do the federal regulations: Massachusetts patients receive a treatment review and evaluation every 90 days for the entire duration of treatment, whereas federal regulations require treatment plans to be updated every quarter only during the first year of treatment and then twice a year thereafter. Finally, Massachusetts mandates strict patient protections in client termination procedures. Patients must be notified in writing of the reasons for proposed termination and of their opportunity to request a hearing to appeal the decision. Hearing procedures are carefully specified in the regulations.

The contract performance standards that were negotiated between the state and providers require each program to have a licensed physician as the medical director (who need not be full-time), and one full-time equivalent (FTE) physician, nurse practitioner, or physician's assistant for the first 300 admissions. For each additional 300 admissions, one FTE nurse or physician's assistant is required. Medication dispensing must be performed by a registered nurse, a licensed practical nurse, or a pharmacist. An average of 26 urine screens must be performed on each client annually and urine collection must be supervised by a health aide or health care professional.

SUMMARY

The treatment system, as described in this chapter, includes a large number of treatment programs, a complex treatment financing system, and variety of state substance abuse authorities. This system is characterized by regional variation and the absence of data about key questions, such as the number and size of for-profit providers, which have increased more rapidly in recent years than not-for-profit treatment programs.

The effects of federal block grant funding of substance abuse treatment on reducing the availability of data about methadone treatment, for example, as well as the effects of a governmentwide reduction in data collection in the

1980s on substance abuse in general and methadone treatment in particular, create problems for policy makers.

The recommendations of the next chapter, which propose to reduce the scope of federal administrative discretion over treatment programs in favor of greater clinical discretion, informed by clinical practice guidelines, are, the committee believes, quite sound. Their application to all treatment programs would be assisted by the availability of better data.

REFERENCES

Anglin, MD, and McGlothlin. 1985. Methadone maintenance in California: A decade's experience. In: L. Brill, C. Winick, (eds.), *The Yearbook of Substance Use and Abuse* Vol. 3. New York: Human Sciences Press.

Ball, JC, and Ross, A. 1991. *The Effectiveness of Methadone Maintenance Treatment: Patients, Programs, Services, and Outcomes.* New York: Springer-Verlag.

Batten H. et al. 1992. Drug Services Research Survey Final Report: Phase II Contract number 27-1908-319/1. Submitted to the National Institute on Drug Abuse (February 12).

Batten H. et al. 1993. Drug Services Research Survey Revised Final Report: Phase I Non-Correctional Facilities. Contract number 27-1908-319/1. Submitted to the National Institute on Drug Abuse (February 22).

Bureau of the Census. 1993. *Statistical Abstract of the United States.* Washington, D.C.: U.S. Government Printing Office.

D'Aunno, T, and Vaughn, T. 1992. Variations in methadone treatment practices. *Journal of the American Medical Association* 267(2)

Department of Health and Human Services. 1991. *NDATUS Instruction Manual.* DHHS Publication No. (ADM) 91-1838. Rockville, Md.: Alcohol, Drug Abuse and Mental Health Administration.

Department of Health and Human Services. 1993a. *Approval and Monitoring of Narcotic Treatment Programs: A Guide on the Roles of Federal and State Agencies.* (Draft) Contract No. 27-091-004. Washington, D.C.: DHHS.

Department of Health and Human Services. 1993b. *Levo-ALPHA-Acetyl-Methadol (LAAM) in Maintenance; Revision of Conditions for Use in the Treatment of Narcotic Addiction.* No. 58(137). Washington, D.C.: DHHS.

Department of Health and Human Services. 1993c. *National Drug and Alcoholism Treatment Unit Survey (NDATUS): 1991 Main Findings Report.* DHHS Publication No. (SMA) 93-2007. Washington, D.C.: DHHS.

Department of Health and Human Services. 1993d. *State Resources and Services Related to Alcohol and Drug Abuse Problems, Fiscal Years 1987, 1988, 1989, 1990, 1991.* DHHS Publication No. (SMA) 93-1989. Washington, D.C.: DHHS.

Department of Health and Human Services. 1993e. *Substance abuse prevention and treatment block grants.* Federal Register, Vol. 58, No. 60, March 31.

Department of Veterans Affairs. 1993. *Annual Cost Distribution Report for FY 1993.* Washington, D.C.: U.S. Government Printing Office.

Department of Veterans Affairs. 1991. *Annual Report of the Secretary of Veterans Affairs: Fiscal Year 1991.* Washington, D.C.: U.S. Government Printing Office.

Food and Drug Administration. 1993. *Narcotic Treatment Programs Directory.* Rockville, Md.: FDA, Regulatory Management Branch.

General Accounting Office. 1990. *Methadone Maintenance: Some Treatment Programs Are Not Effective; Greater Federal Oversight Needed.* GAO/HRD90-104. Washington, D.C.: U.S. Government Printing Office.

Goldstein, H. 1991. *The Effectiveness of Methadone Maintenance Treatment. Drug Abuse Information and Monitoring Project, California Department of Alcohol and Drug Programs,* White Paper Series 8. Sacramento, CA.

Goldstein, HM. 1989. *The Availability of Methadone Maintenance in California: April 1989.* Part II of a report to the California Department of Alcohol and Drug Programs. Drug Abuse Information and Monitoring Project, White Paper Series 9. Sacramento, CA.

Health Care Financing Administration. 1991. *Medicaid: A Brief Summary of Title XIX of the Social Security Act.* Baltimore: HCFA.

Horgan, C, Larson, MJ, and Simon, L. *Medicaid Funding for Drug Abuse Treatment: A National Perspective.* NIDA Treatment Services Research Monograph, Rockville, Md. forthcoming.

Institute of Medicine. 1990. *Treating Drug Problems.* D. Gerstein and H. Harwood (eds.). Washington, D.C.: National Academy Press.

Kirn, T. 1988. Methadone maintenance treatment remains controversial even after 23 years of experience. *The Journal of the American Medical Association* 260(20): 2970–2975.

Merlis, M. 1993a. *Medicaid: An Overview.* Publication No. 93-144 EPW. Washington, D.C.: The Library of Congress.

Murphy, S, and Rosenbaum, M. 1988. Money for methadone II: Unintended conse quences of limited-duration methadone maintenance. *Journal of Psychoactive Drugs* 20(4).

Norquist, G, Hough, R, Golding, J, and Escobar, J. 1990. Psychiatric disorder in male veterans and nonveterans. *Journal of Nervous and Mental Disease* 178: 328–335.

O'Sullivan, J. 1992. *Medicaid: Eligibility for Families, Children, and Pregnant Women.* Publication No. 93-240 EPW. Washington, D.C.: Library of Congress.

Peterson K, Swindle, R, Paradise M, and Moos R. 1993. *Substance Abuse Treatment Programming in the Department of Veterans Affairs: Staffing, Patients, Services, and Policies.* Palo Alto, Calif.: Program Evaluation Resource Center, Department of Veterans Affairs Medical Center.

Price, R. 1993b. *Medicaid: Eligibility for the Aged, Disabled, and Blind.* Publication No. 93-40 EPW. Washington, D.C.: Library of Congress.

Price, R, Burke, AC, D'Aunno, TA, et al. 1991. Outpatient drug abuse treatment services, 1988: Results of a national survey. In: R. W. Pickens, C. G. Leukefeld, and C. R. Schuster (eds.), *Improving Drug Abuse Treatment.* (NIDA Research Monograph 106, Rockville, Md.: Pp. 63–92.

Schmidt, L, and Weisner, C. 1993. Developments in alcoholism treatment. In: M. Galanter (ed.), *Recent Developments in Alcoholism, Vol. 11: Ten Years of Progress*. New York: Plenum Press.

Solloway, M. 1992. *A Fifty-State Survey of Medicaid Coverage of Substance Abuse Services*. Intergovernmental Health Policy Project. Washington, D.C.: George Washington University.

Vocci, FJ and Sorer, H. 1992. Pharmacotherapies for treatment of opioid dependence. *Journal of Health Care for the Poor and Underserved* 3:109–124.

7

Treatment Standards and Optimal Treatment

As discussed in chapter 1, the rationale for government policy in opiate addiction treatment, in the view of the committee, flows from concerns for the functioning of individual addicts, the minimization of public health risks, and the reduction of criminal behavior associated with drug abuse, as well as the minimization of methadone diversion consistent with these objectives.

Although the Secretary of Health and Human Services is obligated under the law to set standards for narcotic addiction treatment, and the federal methadone regulations have been the sole means for implementing this requirement historically. The committee views one major purpose of standards to be improving the quality of treatment. In this chapter, we consider how standards should be implemented to improve treatment.

We begin by discussing the definition of terms, we then consider the characteristics of good treatment with respect to patient evaluation and admission, maintenance pharmacotherapy, medically supervised withdrawal, inpatient treatment, and pain management. As the discussion of our topics unfolds, we have occasion to refer to the barriers to effective treatment and suggest specific changes that should be made in the current regulations to remove or minimize these barriers. Throughout, we distinguish between methadone as a medicine and methadone maintenance treatment as a program of comprehensive services that enhance the effectiveness of the pharmacological treatment.

The detailed discussion in this chapter of treatment in relation to the federal methadone regulations stems from the view of the committee that regulations have an appropriate place, but that they can be improved in a number of ways. Moreover, improvements lie in the direction of reducing governmental involvement in the regulation of treatment services and relying more on the judgment of clinicians, aided by the development of clinical practice guidelines.

185

The implementation of standards by regulations is not, in fact, required by the statute. Nonetheless, the regulations have been relied on to prescribe standards which have discouraged the development of alternative or complementary approaches. Chapter 8, therefore, deals with the role of federal regulations in improving treatment, as well as other ways to implement standards, such as clinical practice guidelines and formal quality assurance systems, and with issues of federal government leadership.

DEFINITION OF TERMS

The following definitions are put forward to clarify certain important concepts. *Tolerance* is the condition resulting from continued use of an opiate drug (or of any substance) that makes it necessary to use increasing amounts of the drug to produce the desired effect. *Physical dependence* is the condition resulting from repeated administration of a drug that necessitates its continued use to prevent the unpleasant withdrawal syndrome that occurs when the drug is abruptly discontinued. Although physical dependence is associated with tolerance, the latter can occur without causing physical dependence. *Addiction* is a condition characterized by lack of control and compulsion that lead to illicit or inappropriate drug-seeking behavior. It can occur with or without physical dependence. An *opiate agonist* is a drug that mimics the effects of endorphin, a naturally occurring compound, thus producing an opiate effect by interaction with the opioid receptor site. Examples are morphine, heroin, and methadone. An *opiate antagonist* is a drug that displaces any opiate agonists and binds with the opioid receptor, thereby inhibiting the opiate effect of the agonist drug. An example is naloxone or naltrexone (Trexan), which prevents or reverses the effects of heroin by competitive binding at the receptor site. *Opiate agonist pharmacotherapy* refers to therapy based on a drug action that mimics the effects of another opiate drug. An example is the therapeutic use of methadone, an opiate agonist used to treat opiate addiction. *Opiate antagonist pharmacotherapy* involves the use of a drug that inhibits or prevents the effects of opiate agonist drugs. An example is the therapeutic use of naltrexone to block the effects of heroin or other opiate agonist drugs.

The two primary clinical applications of opiate agonist pharmacotherapy to treat opiate addiction are the limited-term withdrawal of an addict from opiate use with the objective of achieving abstinence from illicit opiates and other psychoactive substances (known as detoxification treatment) and chronic administration of medication for chronic opiate addiction (known as maintenance treatment).

These terms—"detoxification treatment" and "methadone maintenance treatment"—raise several issues. "Detoxification" has posed the most difficulty.

In the 1950s, at the Lexington Public Health Hospital, methadone was used as a way to "detoxify" heroin addicts by substituting methadone for heroin, then tapering the dose to zero to minimize withdrawal symptoms. The term "detoxification" entered the regulations in 1972 and was incorporated into the Narcotic Addict Treatment Act (NATA) in 1974. The term has been used historically to mean the use of methadone to terminate opiate use through the reduction of the methadone dose, and then to terminate methadone use as well.

Current regulations, based on the NATA, specify short-term (up to 30 days) and long-term (31 to 180 days) detoxification treatment. The original 1972 regulations limited detoxification to 21 days and made no distinction between short and long term. Three problems exist with these arbitrarily defined treatment periods. First, they bear no documented relationship to scientific or clinical data. Rather, they are based on a philosophic commitment to a drug-free state that ignores such data. Second, they arbitrarily constrain treatment decisions by clinicians. Third, treatment based on these artificial time limits often results in the patient relapsing to illicit opiate use. "Such" limits defeat the ultimate purpose that detoxification treatment was designed to serve, namely, of using methadone to withdraw from *both* the use of illegal opiates, such as heroin, *and* from continued reliance on methadone itself.

Clinical experience of more than two decades has thus shown repeatedly that linking treatment to these predetermined time periods for "detoxification" does not help chronically relapsing opiate-dependent patients to recover from their addiction. Rather, these arbitrary periods may actually hinder recovery by encouraging treatment decisions based on nonclinical, administrative grounds. For example, because patients admitted for "detoxification" represent a short-term obligation of treatment programs, by definition, they often receive fewer services than patients admitted for maintenance, without respect to clinical need. Not surprisingly, the results of detoxification treatment have been generally disappointing. High rates of relapse to drug use and abuse have been a frequent correlate of detoxification treatment (Lipton and Maranda, 1981; Resnik, 1983. The steady lengthening of the permissible treatment period over time and the differentiation of detoxification into short- and long-term treatment is tacit recognition by the government of these disappointing results.

Therefore, the committee recommends that "medically supervised withdrawal (MSW)" be substituted for "detoxification" and be defined as follows: "Acute or short-term (several days, several weeks, or a few months) administration of an approved, long-acting opiate agonist drug to an individual patient, at a steadily reduced dose on a schedule and rate such that the individual is able to continue to function with a tolerable level of discomfort and the use of short-acting opiates by the individual is discouraged."

With respect to the term "methadone maintenance treatment," the committee also proposes that the definition of the sustained use of methadone to treat opiate addiction in the regulations be modified to describe the treatment more accurately.

Specifically, the committee recommends that "maintenance pharmaco-therapy (MPT)" be substituted for "methadone maintenance" (at Sec. 291.505(a)(2)) of the regulations and be defined as follows: "Sustained administration of an approved opiate agonist drug, at relatively stable doses, for the treatment of opiate addiction."

In addition, the committee proposes that the following language changes be made in the regulations and incorporated in any practice guidelines that are developed later:

Replace all references to the treatment of "narcotic addicts" with references to the treatment of "opiate addiction"; replace all references to "narcotic dependence" with "opiate addiction"; and replace all references to "opiate addict" with the definition of "opiate addiction." "Opiate" defines the class of drug in question; "narcotic" refers to any stupor-inducing drug, and is a legal term that includes cocaine (see chapter 5). "Addiction" is to be distinguished from "dependence."
Replace the term "continuous or sustained use of a narcotic drug" (at Sec. 291.505 (a)(1)), and wherever it is used which could refer to pain patients, **with the term "addiction to opiates."**
Eliminate the definition of "narcotic dependent" (Sec. 291.505(a)(5)), which fails to define the class of drugs and could be confused with physical dependence on nonopiate drugs.
Replace the term "narcotic treatment program" (Sec. 291.505(a)(6)), with the term "opiate addiction treatment program." Narcotic is an inappropriate adjective for "treatment program," and the greater specificity of the latter term is desirable.
Replace all references to the treatment of "narcotic addicts with a narcotic drug" with references to the treatment of "opiate addiction with an opiate." The greater specificity of the latter terms is desirable.
Replace all references to the term "physiological dependence" with the term "physical dependence" and eliminate any use of "dependence" as a synonym for "addiction." "Physical" has a clear meaning; "physiological" does not change the meaning but does not add clarity. "Dependence" and "addiction" are to be distinguished; the former can occur without the latter.

PATIENT EVALUATION AND ADMISSION CRITERIA

The evaluation of patients for admission to treatment is relatively simple at the two ends of the spectrum defined by long-term methadone maintenance and detoxification. Opiate addicts whose addiction has persisted over many years and who have a history of multiple relapses should typically be admitted to maintenance treatment. Individuals with only a brief history of opiate use (of a few weeks or months) who have developed tolerance and physical dependence and cannot stop use on their own are likely candidates for detoxification.

The cases that do not fall clearly in either category pose the greatest challenge to the clinician. When the assessment of a candidate patient is not immediately clear, evaluation and admission decisions should be made by well-trained clinicians in consultation with the patient. The current federal methadone regulations do not help the clinical assessment of patients. Rather, they specify formulas, such as minimum standards for admission, which have no clinical relevance for determining which patients are eligible for maintenance and which for detoxification.

In general, the decision to admit a patient to methadone pharmacotherapy, either medically supervised withdrawal,(MSW) or maintenance pharmacotherapy (MPT), should be based on a comprehensive evaluation and a clear clinical diagnosis of physical opiate dependence and chronic opiate addiction, defined to include the psycho-social-behavioral characteristics described as "drug-seeking behavior." A comprehensive evaluation should establish patient eligibility for methadone pharmacotherapy on the basis of the following: current physical opiate dependence and addiction; objective findings and subjective reports of the patient that support the need for pharmacotherapy; a judgment that the patient is capable of understanding and participating in a treatment program; and an expressed willingness of the patient to enter treatment after the nature of that treatment has been carefully explained to him or her.

Once a primary diagnosis of opiate addiction has been made, an assessment of its duration and severity should determine the most appropriate treatment for the patient. The decision to treat should consider all available treatments, including nonpharmacological interventions.

The initial assessment must also address the other medical and psychosocial needs of prospective patients needs. These are likely to be considerable in the case of candidates for MPT, since most such patients have diverse and often severe medical and psychological needs that require attention independently of the addiction treatment decision.

It is essential to obtain informed patient consent to treatment at the initiation of treatment and again when the patient is stabilized. Obtaining consent should include a thorough explanation of clinic rules and procedures and the patient's acknowledgment that these have been explained and understood. Patient consent should be periodically reviewed.

Admission to Medically Supervised Withdrawal

The determination of who should be placed on MSW is based on whether the individual has an acute or chronic addiction, is or is not eligible for MPT, and prefers MSW to MPT. The patients for whom MSW is appropriate are the following:

1. An individual diagnosed as having acute opiate addiction and who is ineligible for MPT. Although ineligible for MPT, the patient prefers MSW to an arbitrarily defined detoxification schedule or to no treatment at all.

2. A chronic opiate addict who wishes to terminate the illicit use of opiates but does not wish to begin a program of MPT, even though he or she may meet the eligibility criteria for MPT, even though he or she may meet the eligibility criteria for MPT.

3. A chronic opiate addict who has experienced the adverse effects of too rapid a reduction of methadone dose under an arbitrarily defined detoxification schedule, and who may have relapsed to the use of illicit opiates, and who wishes to withdraw from methadone use at a slower, less disruptive pace.

4. An MPT patient who wishes to withdraw from methadone use, whose dose may be tapered off on an individualized basis as he or she continues MPT.

5. Patients living in areas where MPT is not available, and who may have to be put on MSW by default.

Individual patient assessments should determine what elements of comprehensive treatment should be in the patient's treatment plan. Although the treatment plan will change to reflect changes in the patient's clinical situation, it should be recognized that the probably shorter-term MSW patient may require more, not less, intensive and comprehensive care than the longer-term MPT patient.

Admission to Maintenance Pharmacotherapy

Admission to methadone maintenance treatment was originally limited to the "hard-core heroin addict," defined as a person with a year or more of daily self-administration of heroin. Current regulations still draw the line at an addiction history of at least one year duration. The *intensity, severity,* and *course* of the addiction history, however, must also be considered in the diagnosis, and not only the literal "history" based on dates provided by an applicant, who is often suffering from withdrawal during the initial interview. In some cases, an individual with as little as six months of heavy heroin use may be diagnosed as chronically opiate-dependent, even though a period of addiction closer to twelve months is needed in most cases.

MPT should be reserved for the chronic cases of opiate addiction, as determined by the full array of clinical diagnostic criteria discussed above (pp. 8–9). The basis for requiring that admission be limited to chronic opiate addiction is that long-term exposure to opiates, including medications such as methadone and LAAM, may result in the adaptation or alteration of some neurobiological function. The patient with chronic opiate addiction is likely to have experienced this process of adaptation or alteration already.

Other factors that should be considered by clinicians in the decision to begin MPT, in addition to current physical dependence on opiates and length of opiate use, include currently approved exceptions in the regulations, such as patients with history of chronic opiate addiction (pregnant women, those recently released from correctional or chronic care facilities, and former MPT patients at risk of relapse).

Proper Patient Placement

Admission to MPT should generally be limited to patients with opiate addiction. Unfortunately, a single clear definition of opiate addiction does not exist. Clinicians working in the field of addiction medicine are clear that opiate physical dependence alone does not equal opiate addiction. In addition to opiate physical dependence, addiction requires loss of control resulting in continued use of opiates despite adverse consequences. Loss of control may be characterized as illicit or inappropriate drug seeking behavior, even in the absence of pain or withdrawal.

Some members of the committee are concerned that distinctions between opiate addiction and opiate physical dependence may not be adequate to prevent inappropriate admissions to long-term MPT. For example, chronic pain patients who become physically dependent on opiates and then experience withdrawal symptoms when opiates are reduced or discontinued are sometimes referred, inappropriately, to methadone treatment programs which treat opiate addiction.

The pain patient, whose remission of pain allows discontinuance of opiates, often requires treatment for opiate withdrawal symptoms. However, these patients usually manifest no compulsion or drug-seeking behavior. The treatment of pain patients who do not have a diagnosis or history of opiate addiction in the setting of a program designed for the treatment of opiate addiction is rarely appropriate. Such pain patients are more appropriately managed in the pain clinic or in a physician's office. On the other hand, some methadone treatment programs may be well-equipped to deal with pain patients, especially those located in hospitals.

Two Conclusions

The committee draws two conclusions from the above discussion about patient evaluations. First, the assessment of opiate addiction should be based on clinical diagnostic criteria and should not be determined by formulas set forth in regulations. Second, the diagnostic criteria for MPT should be set forth in clinical practice guidelines, such as the CSAT State Methadone Treatment Guidelines (see, e.g., Center for Substance Abuse Treatment, 1992) or the American Society of Addiction Medicine criteria, (see ASAM, 1991). Such guidelines should indicate the level of training and competence that is desirable for clinicians in treatment programs authorized to make such a diagnosis.

Therefore, the IOM committee recommends that the regulations acknowledge the importance of the clinical evaluation of patients and minimize the administrative criteria in the maintenance pharmaco-therapy admission decision by (1) noting that opiate physical dependence alone is not sufficient grounds for recommending MPT; (2) substituting "medically supervised withdrawal (MSW)" for "detoxification" and substituting "maintenance pharmacotherapy (MPT)" for "methadone maintenance"; and (3) removing all language that encourages or discourages either MSW or MPT on the basis of nonclinical criteria (e.g., admission criteria that include arbitrary time frames.)

MAINTENANCE PHARMACOTHERAPY

Effective maintenance treatment for individual patients involves two elements—the provision of an appropriate dose of medication and a range of comprehensive services. The level of each of these elements is expected to change as a function of time in treatment and the patient's needs. We deal first with dosing principles, then with comprehensive services. In addition, we discuss take-home medication and urine testing. Implications for regulation are then examined, followed by a concluding subsection on addiction in pregnant women.

Dosing

The goals for pharmacotherapy of addiction to opiates include the following: the prevention or reduction of withdrawal symptoms, the prevention or reduction of drug craving, the prevention of relapse to use of such drugs, and, when possible, the restoration or movement toward normality of any physiological functions disrupted by chronic drug abuse (Kreek, 1992). Effective opiate pharmacotherapy (methadone or LAAM) is achieved by a dosage level that establishes a "steady-state" occupation of adequate numbers of specific opioid receptors.

Dosing can be divided into phases (Payte and Khuri, 1992), which are indicated on Table 7-1. The committee concludes that dosing practices should not be determined by regulations but instead should be based on current scientific and clinical knowledge and on published guidelines, where feasible. What that knowledge tells us is:

1. Patients tend to vary in level of opioid tolerance and dependence as well as in the absorption, metabolism, and elimination of methadone. Hence it is essential to determine each dose individually, taking patient reports seriously and monitoring the patient's reaction to medication carefully. In the patient with established tolerance to opiates the initial dose of methadone is usually 20 to 40 mg. The purpose of the initial and first few doses is to relieve withdrawal signs and symptoms that are present. The dose required to accomplish this purpose varies according to the level of tolerance and dependence. A single dose of methadone reaches a blood level peak between 2 and 4 hours. It is prudent to wait at least 3–4 hours before additional doses of methadone are provided and important that patients be observed closely in the induction period at the initiation of treatment. Abstinence symptoms may appear before the end of this initial, 24-hour dosing interval, because there has been no accumulation of methadone in the liver and other tissues to sustain steady drug levels in the circulation. Therefore, additional small doses of methadone (5–20 mg) may be needed three to twelve hours after the initial dose, for up to one week, to prevent signs and symptoms of opiate withdrawal (Dole et al., 1966; Kreek, 1991c; Payte and Khuri, 1992).

2. After initial dosing, the goal is to achieve full prevention of both signs and symptoms of withdrawal for 24 hours. The 24-hour period requires that a steady-state level be established, which may require 5–10 days. Assessment of the effectiveness of dose in the first few days is best determined by the res-

TABLE 7-1 Principles of Methadone Pharmacotherapy Dosing

Phase	Purpose	Dose (range, mg)
Initial dose	Relieve withdrawal symptoms	20–40 in tolerant patients
Early induction	Bring dose to established tolerance level	5–10 mg every 3-24 hours
Late induction	Assure adequacy of dose; "blockade"	+/– 5–10 mg every 7 days
Maintenance/ Stabilization	Achieve goals listed above	60–120 mg, could be more, or less
Long-term mainte- nance or medical maintenance	Maintain stability and physiologic normalcy	60–120 mg
Medically supervised withdrawal	Gradual reduction of tolerance to zero	Variable, reductions of 10% of dose level every 7–10 days (as tolerated)

ponse at 10–12 hours after the dose, rather than at 24 hours. Early in treatment, the patient may need more *time* on the same dose of methadone rather than a larger dose of methadone. After initial stabilization, daily doses of methadone are then gradually increased, by 5 or 10 mg each week, until a full treatment dose of 60 to 120 mg is reached by the end of an induction period of four to eight weeks.

3. In addition to prevention of the withdrawal syndrome, the dose should reduce or eliminate drug hunger or craving. Given the substantial availability of opiates in the environment of many patients, those individuals who may be vulnerable to the opportunistic use of opiates should have their dose gradually raised to a "blockade" level. The resulting cross-tolerance will ensure that supplemental opiates will not produce the desired effect. For most patients the "blockade" level will be between 60 and 120 mg daily. Some patients do well on less than 60 mg and others may require more than 120 mg (Dole, 1989; Inturrisi and Verebey, 1972; Kreek, 1973; Loimer, Schmit, et al., 1991).

4. Determining methadone blood levels is seldom necessary but may be helpful to ensure adequate patient dosing in those situations where patients experience problems on doses that are usually in the therapeutic range. Blood levels should remain at levels greater than 150 ng/ml. An optimum level of methadone will be based on a clinical judgment of the ability of the patient to abstain from heroin and other opiates, and the comfort level of the patient. Optimal individual doses are more likely in the 400 ng/ml range. It is recommended that blood be collected at 3–4 hours and again at 24 hours after an observed dose (Payte and Khuri, 1992). The rate of elimination is as important as the actual levels. The peak should be no more than twice that of the trough level. Rapid metabolizers may benefit from split doses. (See chapter 2.)

5. Stable maintenance doses may require adjustments from time to time. The vast majority of dose determinations can be based purely on clinical signs and symptoms. Subjective reports of the patients must be heeded as it is not realistic to rely solely on objective evidence for dose adjustments, especially when a patient is experiencing drug hunger or cravings. At the same time, the clinician must be alert to the occasional patient who wants a higher dose than necessary in order to sell a portion of it "on the street."

6. Pregnant patients are managed by the same principles but with some special considerations (see below).

In light of the above, the committee recommends that the regulations retain the language that "the amount of the initial dose should not exceed 30 mg" in order to protect the safety of the newly admitted methadone patient. Other dosing restrictions should be removed from the regulations, including the language that "the administering physician shall ensure that a daily dose greater than 100 mg is justified in the patient record"; patient take-home medication and other clinic privileges should not be contingent on dose levels, and clinical practice guidelines should be developed to assist clinicians regarding adequate dosing and take-home practices.

Comprehensive Treatment Services

Methadone as a medication is but one element of a comprehensive treatment program offering a full range of services, which include methadone administration, counseling, and other medical care (Hubbard et al., 1989; McLellan et al., 1993; TOPS 1979-1981).

The premise of this argument is that the overriding goal of MPT is to *habilitate* (to make capable, to qualify) and *rehabilitate* (to return to a former capacity, healthy condition, or useful function) patients with opiate problems to a basic level of social, life, work, and health capabilities that help them become productive, independent members of society.

Opiate-dependent patients typically have a range of medical, psychological, economic, legal, and social problems. For example, studies by Rounsaville et al. (1982), Khantzian and Treece (1985) and Woody et al. (1983) have documented the high proportion of psychiatric diagnoses seen in methadone maintained patients. Ball and Nurco, among others, have shown very high rates of individual and property crime among opiate-dependent patients. Metzger and Platt (1988) have shown the extreme problems of unemployment and deficits in job-seeking skills among a significant proportion of these patients. Studies by Stanton and his colleagues (Stantan, 1979; Stanton et al., 1992) have documented the serious family and relationship problems found in opiate-dependent patients maintained on methadone. Finally, the problems of AIDS, hepatitis, tuberculosis, and other infectious diseases are widely documented and growing rapidly among opiate-dependent patients.

It is important to note that these problems, rather than opiate use itself, are the major sources of concern to society. These "associated problems" are not only a source of substantial direct expense to the country but are in turn associated indirectly with the apparent deterioration in the quality of life for many areas of the country. Thus, while methadone maintenance can be seen as a service to or even a privilege for the affected individual because it reduces his/her withdrawal symptoms and cravings for opiates, to the extent that it is effective in reducing the social harm caused by these associated problems, methadone maintenance treatment may be seen as a public health benefit to society, similar to education and vaccination programs. It must be emphasized that the potential benefits to the public derive from reductions in the associated problems of crime, loss of productivity, and disproportionate use of medical and social services for those in methadone treatment—and not from reductions in the use of opiates per se.

Although these associated problems occur disproportionately among opiate-abusing patients, there has been debate about their origins and the appropriate role of methadone maintenance treatment in addressing them. If these additional problems were due entirely or even predominantly to the use of opiates, and if the methadone medication by itself were effective in eliminating opiate use, then the provision of methadone alone would likely be effective both in reducing the target problem of opiate use and in bringing about the larger social goals of rehabilitation. It is well documented that methadone *in adequate doses, by itself,* can produce marked reductions in illicit opiate use (Yancovitz, DesJarlais, et al., 1991; McLellan, Woody, et al. 1988). Further, it seems clear that these reductions in illicit opiate use as well as the accompanying stabilization of craving is a necessary precondition for achieving any additional rehabilitation.

Current practice in most methadone maintenance programs includes, at best, an evaluation of a newly admitted patient's medical and psychosocial treatment problems, followed by assignment to a paraprofessional "counselor," who often has a 50-patient caseload. During the course of treatment over succeeding weeks and even years, the counselor—not professionally trained physicians, social workers, or pscyhotherapists—is typically the only treatment provider available to or seen by the patient. Even patients with very serious medical, social and psychiatric problems often receive no more than the usual paraprofessional, drug-focused counseling during methadone treatment. Such counseling is a form of advice and general support, usually delivered by an individuals with substantial field experience but rarely having advanced training in social work, psychology, nursing, or medicine. The major focus of drug counseling is on monitoring drug use by reviewing urinalysis reports, monitoring problematic behaviors, encouraging compliance with clinic rules, helping to resolve acute social or personal crises, encouraging patients to seek and maintain gainful employment, providing (where possible) liaison services with physicians, courts, and social agencies, and encouraging patients to talk about important personal or family problems.

Several studies document the efficacy of this form of treatment service for the "average" methadone maintained patient. At the same time, this mainstay of methadone maintenance treatment is frequently in short supply due to large patient caseloads (current regulations allow for caseloads of 50 patients per counselor). More importantly, it is clear from numerous studies that patients with more severe medical, psychiatric, employment, housing, and legal problems are not adequately served by drug counseling alone. There is accumulating evidence that even adequate doses of methadone, in the absence of additional counseling and medical and social services, *produce suboptimal reductions in opiate use* and have only minimal effects on reducing other drug and/or alcohol problems of these patients or solving their health, economic, crime, and medical problems that are so important to society (McLellan, Woody, et al., 1988; Ball and Ross, 1991).

Further, it is clear that the presence of these associated problems significantly affects the course and overall results of treatment (Hubbard and Marsden, 1986; Sells, Demarre, et al., 1986; McLellan, Luborsky, et al., 1982; McLellan, Luborsky, et al., 1986). Patients in methadone maintenance who have had little improvement in their employment, family, and psychiatric problems will be in greater danger of relapse.

Over the past 10 years numerous investigations have evaluated the benefits obtained by adding professional interventions to basic methadone maintenance. For example, in an initial investigation of the "active ingredients" of treatments McLellan et al. (1988) evaluated the contribution of drug counseling services to overall outcome from methadone maintenance. The drug counselor assignment was found to be a particularly significant aspect of methadone maintenance treatment. Woody et al. (Woody, McLellan, et al., 1987; Woody, McLellan, et al., 1984) have shown the benefits of adding professional psychotherapy to methadone maintenance, while Metzger and Platt have shown similar benefits from adding employment and skills training.

A more recent study of different *levels of services* within a methadone maintenance treatment program goes directly to the question of the minimal conditions necessary for social rehabilitation and the effects of adding counseling and other services to methadone maintenance (McLellan, Woody, et al., 1988). In that study three groups of voluntary patients were randomly assigned at the beginning of their methadone maintenance treatment to receive different types and amounts of treatment services. All patients received initial physical examinations, laboratory testing, and a short program of AIDS education. Thereafter, level one patients received *methadone maintenance (blocking doses of 60 mg. or more) without additional counseling* except in an emergency basis. Level two patients received the same *methadone stabilization plus regular counseling* by a trained rehabilitation specialist, but no additional services. Level three patients received the same services as level two patients, but in addition were *also provided family therapy, employment, counseling, and regular medical and psychiatric care* on an as-needed basis at the methadone program site.

There were significant differences in the amounts of improvement shown across these three levels. Patients in Level One showed some improvement in their opiate use but not in their cocaine use or in any of their other problems. They also showed minor improvements in employment, but no other changes. The simple addition of a counselor to this level of services (ie. Level Two) was associated with enhanced improvement in many problem areas, but adding services of family therapists, physicians and social workers for Level Three patients produced still greater changes, particularly among the most severely impaired patients. In summary, this work indicates that counseling and especially professional interventions *should be added* to standard methadone treatment and *these interventions can produce significant improvements* in drug use, employment, legal status, and health services utilization in individuals with multiple problems.

Three conclusions flow from existing research on the rehabilitative goals of methadone maintenance treatment. First, the available national data indicate that opiate-dependent patients at the time of treatment admission *typically show a wide range of serious health and social problems in addition to their primary problem of opiate dependence.*

Second, data from three decades of controlled clinical trials and field research indicate that these opiate-dependent patients show *improvement in, if not elimination of, their opiate addiction with the provision of adequate doses of methadone.* This improvement, in turn, tends to result in reductions in opiate-related crime and in the direct effects of opiate use such as needle sharing (e.g., in transmission of AIDS and other infectious diseases).

Third, *improvements in the important social and self-support areas are at least in part related to the types and amounts of counseling and other professional medical and social services provided during treatment.* There is little evidence that, at least at the initiation of methadone treatment, the provision of methadone *by itself* can lead to reductions in other important problem areas of nonopiate drug use, alcohol dependence, unemployment, psychiatric problems, and disproportionate use of health care services. Data from the past ten years have shown that counseling and particularly professional health care and social services can significantly augment the direct effects of methadone in achieving reductions in opiate use and are essential to achieving the important goals of social rehabilitation for opiate-dependent patients.

Take-Home Medication

The committee discussed at length the issue of take-home medications. It concurs with existing federal regulations providing that "take-home medicine may be given only to a patient who, in the reasonable judgment of the program physician, is responsible in handling narcotic drugs" (21 CFR 291.505(d)(6)(iv) (A)). The committee also believes that decisions about patient take-home medication should be made only by the medical director of the treatment program, and should be documented in the patient's medical chart.

The basis for clinical judgment should continue to be the following eight criteria currently set forth in the federal methadone regulations (see 21 CFR 291.505(d)(6)(iv)(B)): (1) absence of recent abuse of drugs (opiate and nonopiate), including alcohol; (2) regularity of clinic attendance; (3) absence of serious behavioral problems at the clinic; (4) absence of known recent criminal activity, e.g., drug dealing; (5) stability of the patient's home environment and social relationships; (6) length of time in maintenance treatment; (7) assurance that take-home medication can be safely stored within the patient's home; and (8) whether the rehabilitative benefit to the patient derived from decreasing the frequency of clinic attendance outweighs the potential risks of diversion. Clinician decisions should be documented relative to each of these criteria.

A majority of the committee believes that the current regulations are too restrictive regarding the schedule of clinic treatment visits required before take-home medication can be administered and in the maximum permissible take-home supply. They would prefer that regulations read as follows: In the first month of treatment there should be six clinic treatment visits a week, and maximum take-home supply should be limited to a single day; in the second month, there should be at least three clinic treatment visits a week, with a maximum take-home supply of two days; in the third month, patients should visit the clinic for treatment at least twice a week, and be eligible for a maximum take-home supply of three days; in the remaining months of the first year, clinic treatment visits should be weekly at least, with a maximum take-home supply of seven days; after one year, a patient should be eligible for medical maintenance, involving monthly visits and a maximum take-home supply of 31 days. The rationale for this take-home schedule is to permit treatment plans to be tailored more closely to the needs of the individual patient, facilitate the entry into treatment of patients who may be more functional than those "last resort" patients who constitute the great majority of the treated population, and vest more authority for clinical decisions in clinicians.

A minority of the committee, though sympathetic to the above objectives, is reluctant to replace the existing regulations with a more flexible set of rules and to recommend changes designed for the "best" patients and most scrupulous clinicians, which, if adopted, would become the standard for all. The rationale for retaining existing regulations is to pace the progress of patients in relation to reasonable expectations, to minimize opportunity for malpractice by unscrupulous physicians, and to maintain the credibility of treatment programs that could easily suffer from the behavior of a few such individuals.

Urine Testing

Federal regulations now require treatment programs to conduct urine tests of methadone patients at admission, plus a minimum of eight times in the initial year, and quarterly thereafter, except for patients receiving a six-day take-home supply, who must be tested monthly. The committee accepts this requirement as a minimum. State authorities and individual treatment programs sometimes impose stricter urine testing requirements than these.

Urine testing is a helpful clinical tool, useful as a way to determine patient progress and compliance with treatment protocols. It should be used in conjunction with other clinical tools, never as a sole indicator of action.

Implications for Regulations

The above conclusions regarding the habilitation and rehabilitation of patients in methadone and other opiate substitution therapies support recognition and acceptance of the proposition that **the full potential of metha-done maintenance as a significant public health service to society will be realized only if it is financially and professionally supported to the point at which it can offer necessary habilitative and rehabilitative services.** Both a scientific evaluation of existing treatment programs (Woody, et al., 1983; Hubbard and Marsden, 1986) and a inspection of national media stories about methadone make it apparent that the present system of care offered by methadone maintenance programs has deteriorated badly over the past ten to fifteen years while the number, chronicity, and complexity of the problems presented by the patients have increased (e.g., AIDS, TB, cocaine, crime). At this point, the best that is available to even seriously impaired opiate-dependent patients in methadone maintenance is the availability of paraprofes-sional drug counseling. While important and necessary, it is clear that drug counseling alone (especially when compromised by caseloads of 50 patients) is not sufficient to address the serious problems of medical illness, psychopa-thology, dangerous or inadequate living situations and lack of self-support skills, so often presented by these patients. The committee believes that a full range of medical, psychiatric, and social services is needed to achieve the optimal benefits of MPT treatment.

Although the committee believes that additional treatment services are cost-effective, it recognizes that many treatment programs are not now providing them. Moreover, a requirement that they be provided could very well impose an economic burden on many treatment programs that would force them to cease providing services altogether. The committee notes that the fiscal year 1995 budget submission and the recently-enacted urine bill future may result in increased future resources for treatment (see chapter 8). It urges the responsible federal agencies to monitor the flow of funds to treatment programs and to require that comprehensive services be provided as available resources are increased.

Given adequate financial support, regulations could specify that MPT programs provide the following services toward the goal of realizing the full potential of such programs to produce public benefits:

1. *Perform a comprehensive evaluation of the full range of medical, employment, alcohol, criminal, and psychological problems of all patients admitted to methadone maintenance and medically supervised withdrawal.* As indicated above, it is in the public interest for methadone maintenance programs to address the "addiction related" problems of unemployment, crime,and infectious diseases. If these problems are to be addressed effectively, they will have to be evaluated and addressed in the initial treatment plan for all patients.

2. *Offer screening for diseases such as AIDS, tuberculosis, hepatitis, and sexually transmitted diseases on-site or nearby.* These diseases are disproportionately represented in the opiate-abusing population and represent a risk to all society as well as to the individuals directly affected. Typically, few medical screening services are available to these patients outside the methadone maintenance programs and it is in the interests of the patient, and of society, to see that these diseases are recognized and treated.

3. *Offer on-site counseling by competent and appropriately supervised addiction counselors.* It is not clear at this time how much counseling is needed for patients entering treatment or for how long. The majority of patients entering treatment, however, will require several sessions of counseling each week during the first months of stabilization, and this level of counseling intensity should be available as a standard part of MPT. It is also unclear whether a particular set of qualifications is required to optimize counseling efficacy and how individuals can be trained to become effective counselors. At the same time, effective counseling can be evaluated and encouraged through ongoing supervision. Thus experienced professional supervision of counseling staff should be a regular part of MPT.

4. *Offer professional medical, social work, and mental health services, preferably on-site or by referral (through contracted interagency agreements).* These services should not be considered "frills," but rather necessary components for MPT programs to achieve the public benefits that justify their existence. Not all patients will need all of these professional services, but the recognition of those who do need the services will be one of the duties of the admission assessment and the ongoing counseling. It may not be possible or even cost-effective for every program to have on-site professionals representing all the services that will potentially be needed by these patients.

Two points are relevant here, however. First, it has been historically difficult to connect opiate-dependent patients with the services that they so clearly need, even when these services are available. There are problems with motivation, disorganization, discrimination, distrust, and confusion that prevent patients from accessing these services even in the best of conditions. In addition, there are many well-documented incidents in which professional services were denied to methadone-maintained patients merely because of the stigma associated with their condition.

When referrals to other treatment sites are required, it is seldom adequate to provide only a written or telephone referral to the other agency. Effective provision of needed services on a referral basis will usually require contractual arrangements between agencies, close working arrangements between responsible individuals at the programs and agencies, and active follow-up by the referring program to insure that services are delivered.

Therefore, the committee recommends that those services that are most clearly needed by admitted patients (e.g., medical and social work) should be provided on-site by competent, licensed, and appropriately supervised professionals wherever possible and, if necessary, by contractual referral arrangements.

This recommendation can only be put in place when MPT programs are restored to a level of funding and professionalism commensurate with the severity of the disorder(s) toward which they are directed. Without infusion of both financial and professional support, any changes in the regulations will be ineffective in increasing the potential benefit of this therapy.

Opiate Addiction in Pregnant Women

The use of methadone to treat pregnant opiate addicts has, for years, been controversial. Although the benefits of methadone pharmacotherapy in pregnancy, in contrast to continued illicit drug use, have been clearly demonstrated, some issues remain unresolved. Studies are complicated by a multitude of confounding variables (Finnegan, 1991). Nevertheless, the following conclusions can be drawn these studies with respect to methadone pharmacotherapy in perinatal addiction:

1. Comprehensive MPT (LAAM is not yet approved for use in pregnant women), when combined with appropriate prenatal care, can reduce the incidence of obstetrical and fetal complications, in utero growth retardation, and neonatal morbidity and mortality (Finnegan, 1991; Kaltenbach, et al., 1992).
2. There is no reported evidence of any toxic effects of methadone in the woman, fetus, or child, although such evidence has been sought.
3. Withdrawal from methadone treatment is rarely appropriate during pregnancy (Finnegan, 1991; American Society of Addiction Medicine, 1991). Relapse to opiate use occurs in these individuals in the same way as in nonpregnant addicts (Finnegan, 1991).
4. Neonatal withdrawal syndrome may occur in methadone-exposed neonates. Treatment protocols are available to assist in appropriate management (Finnegan, 1986; Finnegan, 1990).
5. Increased doses of methadone may be needed during the late stages of pregnancy. Methadone metabolism increases in some pregnant women, thus decreasing the methadone levels in their blood; an individualized dose increase may then be needed to maintain constant plasma levels and prevent symptoms of withdrawal (Kaltenbach, et al., 1992). There is no consistent correlation

between maternal methadone dose and severity of neonatal withdrawal (Stimmel, et al., 1982-1983).

6. Breast feeding may be encouraged during methadone pharmacotherapy, if not otherwise contraindicated (Kaltenbach, 1992).

7. Multiple longitudinal studies find that methadone-exposed infants score well within normal range of development (Kaltenbach, 1992; Kaltenbach and Finnegan, 1984).

8. Obstacles and barriers to methadone pharmacotherapy for pregnant women with opiate addiction (such as lack of financial resources, waiting lists, procedural delays of admission for treatment, or lack of knowledge about how to treat pregnant opiate addicts safely and humanely), must be removed. Pregnant opiate-addicted women need immediate access to methadone treatment services. Limitations in the federal regulations, along with waiting lists for treatment or geographic inaccessibility, create barriers for the safe and effective treatment of this population.

9. More research is needed on innovative models of treatment, including medically supervised withdrawal during pregnancy with residential care, intensive relapse prevention and monitoring, and high-risk prenatal care. Where appropriate, hospitals, clinics, and individual obstetricians should be permitted to administer methadone to a pregnant opiate addict in collaboration with a licensed MPT program.

In light of the above discussion, the committee recommends that regulations (1) require that programs establish rapid admission procedures to facilitate prompt treatment for pregnant opiate addicts; (2) assure alternative ways to provide maintenance treatment for pregnant opiate addicts where treatment is not otherwise available; and (3) allow providers to give maintenance pharmacotherapy outside of a licensed narcotic treatment program. Alternatives to treatment programs might include hospital, pharmacy, clinic, and individual practitioner's office acting as MPT programs for the purpose of prescribing methadone to pregnant opiate addicts who are awaiting admission into a licensed program, or for the duration of the pregnancy for patients in geographic areas where there are no licensed programs. In such cases, the determination of dosage, the treatment plan, and the acceptable time of treatment after conclusion of the pregnancy should be made in consultation with addiction treatment experts and should operate according to specific guidelines for such patients.

MEDICALLY SUPERVISED WITHDRAWAL

As a consequence of the limits of detoxification treatment, discussed earlier, the committee is proposing that the regulations be changed by eliminating the term "detoxification treatment" and replacing it with the term "medically supervised withdrawal." This section outlines the principles of medically supervised withdrawal (MSW), the goal of which is the gradual reduction of the methadone dose to zero at a tolerable rate that neither creates undue discomfort for the patient nor results in his or her relapse to illicit opiate use. Too high a dose serves more of a maintenance than withdrawal purpose; too low a dose impairs functioning and may lead to the substitution of other opiates or drugs, including alcohol.

The individuals for whom MSW is appropriate were indicated earlier in this chapter (see "Patient Evaluation and Admission Criteria"). The principles of long-term medically supervised MSW include the following:

1. Any patient being considered for MSW must be physically dependent upon opiates and therefore have an established opiate tolerance level, which is determined by the amount of methadone required to suppress the signs and symptoms of withdrawal. For the MPT patient that level is roughly equal to the daily dose.

Doses that may range slightly above or below the average tolerance level result in no subjective or objective reactions and define a "comfort zone" for the patient. This range is believed to be up to 10 percent +/- of dosage. Any dose reduction within the comfort zone will usually be well tolerated. Dosage and withdrawal schedules must be individualized and be the result of careful clinical judgment

2. When the dose is reduced within the comfort zone, the degree of tolerance begins to adjust to the new dose level over a period of several days. When the tolerance level equals the reduced dose, the process can be repeated. Intervals of 7–10 days are adequate for adjustment to a single-step reduction in most cases. However, some patients will tolerate more rapid reductions, while others will need additional time.

3. The application of this dose reduction principle would result in MSW treatment lasting for years in some cases. Dose decrements of less than 1 mg are not practical useful. Many clinicians use decrements of 2, 2.5, or 5 mg, depending upon the form of methadone used as well as the tolerance level as reflected by the current average methadone dose.

4. Successful MSW is not assured by simple avoidance of withdrawal syndrome. As the methadone is reduced, a point may be reached for some patients at which daily dose is inadequate to provide the desired level of steady-state occupation of adequate numbers of receptor sites, and symptoms

such as drug craving may recur. Many experienced practitioners of methadone maintenance find that there is an individual methadone dosage in some patients, usually between 15 and 50 mg, at which the patient has considerable difficulty making further reductions.

Patients whose initial treatment is MSW and who then resume opiate use during withdrawal should be encouraged to stabilize themselves on methadone before resuming withdrawal. If appropriate, they may wish to consider initiation or resumption of MPT, instead of proceeding with withdrawal.

Individuals who have withdrawn from methadone under medical supervision should be carefully followed by a treatment program and encouraged to participate in an ongoing program of recovery. In the event of relapse or impending relapse, additional therapeutic measures should be used, including, when appropriate, the rapid resumption of agonist pharmacotherapy.

Under certain circumstances, MSW is initiated against a patient's will (e.g., given the certainty of discharge, the patient may elect MSW rather than pursue transfer to another program or facility). When withdrawal from methadone pharmacotherapy is not medically indicated, it is referred to as involuntary administrative withdrawal. The circumstances that justify involuntary administrative termination from treatment usually involve inappropriate behavior that threatens the program's welfare or jeopardizes the safety or health of patients and staff. Involuntary administrative withdrawal should be the course of last resort when it has been determined that methadone MPT (at the particular program) is no longer appropriate and when no alternative placement for the patient is possible. Transfer to another facility should be aggressively pursued (and documented in the patient's record) and is the preferred course for those patients for whom involuntary administrative discharge is indicated. Only if transfer is not possible, and all alternatives have been exhausted, should involuntary withdrawal commence, and it should be medically supervised.

The decision to terminate methadone maintenance treatment has profound implications for a patient and should not be implemented until the conclusion of a hearing and appeal. In cases of involuntary MSW, it is particularly important that the pace of the withdrawal be accomplished safely (according to standards set forth in this report) and as comfortably as possible in order to minimize the patient's chances for relapse to illicit substance abuse. In cases where a patient's immediate departure from the program is imminent, the patient should be transferred to another facility for involuntary MSW.

MSW patients who experience difficulties with small reductions in dose over considerable intervals of time should be considered for inpatient treatment, alternative or additional pharmacotherapy (clonidine, etc.), or in some cases early admission to maintenance pharmacotherapy. These decisions should be weighed carefully to determine the most appropriate action. Given he risks of HIV, hepatitis, STDs, and TB, any decision that increases the ikelihood that the patient will return to the use of street drugs must be taken eriously.

The outcome of MSW is more likely to depend on such factors as personal notivation, patient resources, support systems (especially family), and appropriate comprehensive treatment than on the number of days in the withdrawal schedule.

In light of the above, the committee recommends: (1) that the Narcotic Addict Treatment Act be amended, if necessary, and the regulations changed accordingly, to eliminate the term "detoxification treatment" and replace it with "medically supervised withdrawal (MSW)," [as defined in the "Definition of Terms" section above]; (2) that no time limits be specified for MSW in the revised regulations; (3) that the revised regulations indicate clearly that MSW is not appropriate for all opiate addicts but is an essential treatment that should be available to all who wish such treatment or would benefit from it; and (4) that clinical practice guidelines, based on the above general principles, be developed to assist clinicians in the clinical management of MSW patients, including the determination of appropriate dose schedules for individual patients.

Recent years have seen increased utilization of nonopiate withdrawal egimens involving clonidine, available to methadone programs only under an nvestigational New Drug (IND) protocol, and in some cases accelerated withdrawal using opiate antagonists. It is beyond the scope of this report to cover his material. The reader is referred to references (Senft, 1991; Brewer et al., 988; Gossop, 1988; Kleber, et al., 1988) for more information.

INPATIENT TREATMENT

The foregoing discussion has dealt with opiate-addicted patients treated in he outpatient setting. The federal regulations governing methadone treatment also affect opiate-addicted individuals in the inpatient setting: methadone maintenance patients who are hospitalized for medical or surgical reasons; and opiate addicted individuals *not* in treatment programs who are admitted for imilar reasons.

Maintenance Pharmacotherapy in Hospital Inpatient Settings

Methadone patients who are admitted to hospitals as inpatients, whether for addiction-related reasons or for unrelated medical and surgical reasons, often are mistreated and mismanaged by hospital staff (Payte and Khuri, 1992). Mistreatment may vary from negative attitudes toward the patients by hospital staff to punitive decisions to withhold methadone; mismanagement may involve failing to provide for the adequate treatment of pain (Zweben and Payte, 1990). Consequently, the committee concluded that some guidance to hospital staff is warranted.

Current regulations do not address the issues of inpatient MPT patients beyond providing a means for continued pharmacotherapy. (Most hospitals have a DEA registration, so they are not prohibited from providing methadone from their pharmacy stock.) These issues are most appropriately addressed by guidelines for hospital staff dealing with such patients. Guidelines, in the judgment of the committee, should reflect the following general principles:

1. On admission of a methadone maintenance patient as a hospital inpatient, the hospital staff should notify the patient's treatment program and confirm the individual's enrollment in the treatment program, methadone dose and time and date of last dose.

2. During a methadone maintenance patient's inpatient stay, the hospital staff should ensure the continuity of methadone pharmacotherapy through the hospital's pharmacy or by making arrangement for its supply through th treatment program in the event the hospital does not stock methadone. Hospital staff and physicians should be prohibited from reducing or denying th methadone dose. Any changes in methadone pharmacotherapy should be made only after consultation with the treatment program physician and with the informed consent of the patient.

3. Before discharge, the hospital staff should notify the methadone treatment program of the time of discharge and the time and amount of last dose of methadone to ensure that outpatient pharmacotherapy can be resumed without interruption.

4. If patients are discharged from acute care to continuing care facilities arrangements for continued provision of methadone should be part of the discharge plan.

Inpatients with Untreated Opiate Addiction

Currently, the federal methadone regulations restrict the use of methadone for treating opiate addiction to the following four situations: (1) a licensed "narcotic treatment program"; (2) a licensed, hospital-based, inpatient addiction treatment unit for detoxification from opiate addiction; (3) a hospital, for temporary maintenance or detoxification, when the admission is for an illness other than opiate addiction; and (4) an outpatient setting (hospital, private practice, clinic, or nursing home with a medical director and 24-hour nursing care) in which methadone is administered daily for a maximum of 3 days while the patient awaits admission into a methadone treatment program. The only circumstance in which methadone can be routinely prescribed and administered on an outpatient basis outside of an officially registered "narcotic treatment program" is for the treatment of pain.

The above restrictions may on occasion result in precipitous withdrawal of opiate-addicted patients. Opiate-addicted patients admitted to hospitals with medical illness related or unrelated to illicit injecting drug use who are in need of methadone treatment pose particular problems. Two unfortunate scenarios can occur: (1) admitted methadone patients are not administered methadone for the relief of opiate withdrawal because detoxification would not be completed before discharge; or (2) opiate-addicted inpatients do receive methadone treatment, but are precipitously withdrawn from methadone at discharge because no arrangement have been made for their transfer to an outpatient treatment program or there are insufficient programs to accept them. Although it has been difficult to document accurately the length of waiting lists for methadone treatment programs, it is well-known in the treatment community that waiting lists exist, especially for those patients who do not have financial or insurance resources. Therefore, it is reasonable to assume that a significant number of patients who seek methadone treatment are unable to obtain access to services.

The committee recommends that the following change be made in the regulations to accommodate the needs of hospitalized opiate addicted patients: Patients who meet the criteria for opiate addiction during any inpatient hospital admission may be treated, when appropriate, with methadone to relieve opiate withdrawal. Patients may then be discharged to methadone treatment programs for their continued treatment. If no resources are available for the patient upon discharge, or if a patient is ready for discharge before his or her withdrawal protocol can be completed, a hospital may accommodate such patients by completing the withdrawal protocol on an outpatient basis. For a patient awaiting admission to a licensed "narcotic treatment program," the hospital may maintain the patient on a maintenance dose of methadone until the patient is admitted by the program. In either case, methadone must be administered daily at the facility by staff licensed to handle and administer opiates. Patients shall not be given prescriptions for methadone for this purpose.

PAIN MANAGEMENT

Methadone was approved by the FDA for the treatment of pain on August 13, 1947. As noted in chapter 1, its use in the treatment of opiate addiction has been highly regulated since late 1972. In the course of this study, the committee received communications from representatives of the pain management community indicating that the methadone regulations had created a number of problems, and much confusion, regarding the use of the drug in pain management. The regulations, intended for one purpose, had generated unanticipated, unintended, and undesirable consequences elsewhere.

Although not asked to deal specifically with issues of pain and its clinical management, the committee has concluded that the intersection of the two uses of methadone—for treating opiate addiction and for pain treatment—is of sufficient importance to warrant this discussion. We identify two issues: first, the problems of the non-opiate addicted pain patient; and second, those of the methadone maintenance patient and the "recovering" opiate-dependent patient who also needs pain treatment. Central to these issues is the need to distinguish the pain patient from the opiate-addicted patient.

Non-Opiate-Addicted Pain Patients

The pain patient with no evidence of addiction poses one set of challenges; the patient with opiate addiction and chronic pain, a different set. The important distinction to be made is that tolerance and physical dependence do not equal addiction (see chapter 2 and the section "Definition of Terms" above).

As a disease, addiction is chronic, progressive, relapsing, and often fatal, and it is characterized by compulsion and continued use of the substance despite adverse consequences (loss of control). The patient with opiate addiction will seek drugs in the absence of any pain or withdrawal symptoms.

The pain patient, on the other hand, will develop tolerance to a number of opioid effects and physical dependence on opiates but will not exhibit the illicit or inappropriate drug-seeking behavior. Nor will many pain patients, in the absence of progressive disease, develop tolerance to the analgesic effects of opioids. The typical pain patient who experiences a cure or remission of pain does not experience the compulsion to resume or continue drugs. Portnoy and Payne (1992) cite three studies: in one, of 11,882 inpatients with no prior history of addiction who were administered opiates, only four cases of psychological dependence could be documented; in the second, a survey of 10,000 burn patients, with no prior history of addiction, who were treated with opiates identified no cases of addiction; in the third, of 2,369 pain patients who regularly used opiates for relief of headache, only three were addicted. The treatment of pain and the treatment of opiate addiction may both involve the prescription of methadone. Beyond that, treatment should be totally distinct. For example, it may be appropriate to treat patients with both a chronic pain disorder and opiate addiction in clinics having well-trained staff, especially those that are an integral part of a hospital. However, it is not appropriate to treat a chronic pain patient *as an opiate addict* in a maintenance pharmacotherapy program, regardless of the degree of tolerance, physical dependence, or duration of the prescription of methadone. On the other hand, persons suffering from opiate addiction are unlikely to receive appropriate treatment in pain clinics and, as a general rule, should not be treated for addiction in such clinics. Those MPT patients who also have chronic pain conditions may require *coordinated* treatment in both clinical settings, which sometimes may exist within in a single organization.

The intensity of chronic or intractable pain cannot be measured objectively and, thus, physicians cannot determine clearly its authenticity. On the other hand, there are clear objective criteria for physical dependence. Physicians treating pain may lack the confidence to continue prescribing schedule II opiate analgesics in the absence of a very clear organic or anatomic basis for pain. The uneasy physician may then make an inappropriate referral to methadone pharmacotherapy.

Therefore, the IOM committee proposes that the regulations establish a clear distinction between opiate addiction and dependence and that any guidelines developed for methadone treatment incorporate this distinction. In addition, the committee recommends that the regulations prohibit the admission of a person being treated solely for chronic pain to an opiate addiction treatment program for treatment as an opiate addict.

As David E. Joranson, of the University of Wisconsin Pain Clinic, wrote to the committee (letter, October 25, 1993): "A person who needs a morphine-like drug only for the medical treatment of intractable pain and to prevent withdrawal associated with the treatment of intractable pain is not a narcotic addict and is not eligible for admission to a narcotic treatment program. A practitioner may prescribe, administer, or dispense narcotic drugs including methadone in the course of professional practice to such a person for the treatment of intractable pain."

It is appropriate that pain experienced by opiate-addicted individuals, along with other medical and psychiatric conditions, be treated in the context of a comprehensive methadone treatment program. Pain treatment centers, on the other hand, are prohibited from and should not attempt treatment of opiate addiction involving any form of MPT, unless licensed and approved to do so. This prohibition should not prevent daily use of methadone at adequate doses for pain treatment as well as prevention of withdrawal symptoms.

Methadone Patients

The opiate-addicted patient with a chronic pain condition can challenge the treating clinician. Effective pain management may require an adequate maintenance dose of methadone as a foundation for pain treatment, but may also involve adequate doses of opiates other than methadone. Both conditions require specialized care.

Methadone maintained patients who are being treated for conditions associated with acute moderate-to-severe pain are often denied treatment for pain. This denial is usually based on two misconceptions: first, that any patient taking a daily dose of methadone should derive adequate analgesia from the maintenance dose, and second, that prescribing an additional amount of an opiate agonist would lead to relapse and/or compromise the treatment of the addiction.

Opiate addiction treatment program medical staff must provide guidance to physicians, dentists, and other practitioners to ensure humane treatment of methadone maintained patients being treated for acute pain. Three principles are involved:

1. Continue methadone pharmacotherapy without interruption.

2. Provide adequate doses of appropriate short acting opiate agonist drugs for pain. Owing to cross-tolerance, higher than normal doses of short-acting opiate agonists will be required for relief of pain. Also, for adequate relief of pain, doses may be needed at more frequent intervals (Payte and Khuri, 1992).

3. Antagonist and mixed agonist-antagonist opiate drugs are not to be given because they may produce a serious withdrawal reaction in opiate tolerant individuals.

"Recovering" Opiate and Other Substance Dependent Patients

Recovering patients who experience acute pain and require opiate pain medication are perceived to be at some risk for relapse to substance abuse or addiction. Clinical experience suggests that such relapses occur more frequently when the patient fails to inform the attending physician(s) of a alcohol or other drug history. The risk is minimal in cases in which the clinician has some understanding of addictive disorders and the recovery process in relation to the treatment of pain. Honest communication between the patient and the physician is essential.

The minimal principles of management are:

1. Provide adequate doses of appropriate short-acting opiate agonist drugs.
2. Relief of pain is essential to avoid distrust and manipulation. Medicate generously for the first 24–48 hours for patients hospitalized for injury or surgery. Be thoughtful about PRN medication by anticipating pain where possible, rather than waiting for pain to manifest itself and then preparing medication, thus losing valuable time. Patient-controlled analgesia may be appropriate and effective if opiate tolerance levels are taken into consideration. Prescriptions offered on a specific schedule can be useful for many patients; a schedule avoids requiring the patient to ask for or to decide whether or not he or she needs medication.
3. Change to nonopiate medication as soon as practical.
4. Avoid extensive prescribing for self-administration of any opiate analgesic medications.

CONCLUDING COMMENTS

The federal methadone regulations have been very extensive and highly prescriptive about basically all aspects of treatment of opiate addiction. From 1972 to the present, these regulations have been modified in useful ways as their limiting effects on treatment have become apparent. However, these modifications, adopted in 1980, 1989, and 1993, have not seriously questioned the underlying assumptions of the original regulations.

The committee's recommendations in this chapter reflect the view that wholesale abandonment of the current regulations is neither feasible nor desirable. The regulations do serve some useful purposes, as indicated above. On the other hand, the recommendations propose to reducing the scope of administrative control by FDA and other DHHS agencies over methadone treatment programs. The corollary of reducing governmental discretion over treatment programs is to recommend that increased reliance be placed on clinical practice guidelines, as they are developed, for clinicians and treatment programs. This shift of responsibility from government officials to clinicians, is already under way in some measure and should be extended, as the committee has recommended.

REFERENCES

American Society of Addiction Medicine. 1991. Statement on Methadone Treatment. *American Society of Addiction Medicine.* Washington, D.C.

Ball, JC and Ross, A. 1991. *The Effectiveness of Methadone Maintenance Treatment: Patients, Programs, Services, and Outcomes.* New York:Springer-Verlag.

Brewer, C, Rezae, and H Bailey, C. 1988. Substance Abuse Treatment Programme. Opioid withdrawal and naltrexone induction in 48-72 hours with minimal drop-out using a modification of naltrexone-clonidine technique. *British Journal of Psychiatry* (September) 153:340–343.

Center for Substance Abuse Treatment. 1992. *State Methadone Treatment Guidelines. Treatment Improvement Protocol (TIP)* Series 1. DHHS Publication No. (SMA) 93-1991. Rockville, Md.: U.S. Department of Health and Human Services.

Dole, VP. 1988. Implications of methadone maintenance for theories of narcotic addiction. *Journal of the American Medical Association* 260:3025–3029.

Finnegan, LP. 1986. Neonatal abstinence syndrome: Assessment and pharmacotherapy. In: F. F. Rubaltelli, and B. Granti, (eds.), *Neonatal Therapy: An Update.* New York: Elsevier Science.

Finnegan, LP. 1990. Neonatal abstinence syndrome. In: N.M. Nelson, (ed.), *Current Therapy in Neonatal-Perinatal Medicine.* Philadelphia: B.C. Becker.

Finnegan, LP. 1991. Treatment issues for opioid-dependent women during the perinatal period. *Journal of Psychoactive Drugs* (2):191–201.

Gossop, M. 1988. Drug Dependence and Clinical Research Unit. Clonidine and the treatment of opiate withdrawal syndrome. *Drug and Alcohol Dependence* (July) 21(3):253–259.

Hubbard, RL and Marsden, ME. 1986. Relapse to use of heroin, cocaine and other drugs in the first year after treatment. In *Relapse and Recovery in Drug Abuse.* NIDA Research Monograph 72, Rockville Md.

Inturrisi, CE, and Verebely, K. 1992. The levels of methadone in the plasma in methadone maintenance. *Clinical Pharmacology and Therapeutics* 13:633–637.

Kaltenbach, K and Finnegan, LP. 1984. Developmental outcome of children born to methadone maintained women: A review of longitudinal studies. *Neurobehavior, Toxicology and Teratology* 6(4):271.

Kaltenbach, K, Silverman, N, and Wapner, R. 1993. Methadone maintenance during pregnancy. In: Center for Substance Abuse Treatment. *State Methadone Treatment Guidelines Treatment Improvement Protocol (TIP)* Series 1. DHHS Publication No. (SMA) 93-1991. Rockville, Md.: DHHS. Pp. 85–93.

Khantzian, EJ, and Treece, K. 1985. DSM-III psychiatric diagnosis of narcotic addicts. *Archives of General Psychiatry* (42):1067–1071.

Kleber, HD, Topazian, M, Riordan, CE, and Kosten, T. 1987. Clonidine and naltrexone in the treatment of heroin withdrawal. *American Journal of Drug and Alcohol Abuse* 13:1–7.

Kreek, MJ. 1973. Plasma and urine levels of methadone. *New York State Journal of Medicine* 73(23):2773–2777.

Kreek, MJ. 1992. Rationale for maintenance pharmacotherapy of opiate dependence. In: O'Brien, CP, and Jaffe, JH, eds. *Addictive States* New York: Raven Press, Ltd. 205–230.

Lipton, DS, and Maranda, NJ. 1981. Detoxification from heroin dependency: An overview of method and effectiveness. *Advances in alcohol and Drug Abuse* 2(1):31–53.

Loimer, N, Schmid, R, Grunberger, J, et al. 1991. Psychophysiological reaction in methadone maintenance patients do not correlate with methadone plasma levels. *Psychopharmacology* (Berl) 103(4):538–540.

McLellan, AT, Arndt, IO, Alterman, AL, Woody GE, Metzger D. 1993. Psychosocial services in substance abuse treatment: A dose-ranging study of psychosocial services. *Journal of the American Medical Association* 269:1953–1959.

McLellan, AT, Woody, GE, Luborsky L, and O'Brien, CP. 1988. Is the counselor an "Active ingredient" in substance abuse treatment? *Journal of Nervous and Mental Disease* 176(7):423–430.

McLellan, AT, Luborsky, L, and O'Brien, CP. 1986. Alcohol and drug abuse in three different populations: Is there improvement and is it predictable? *American Journal of Drug and Alcohol Abuse* 12(2):101–120.

McLellan, AT, Luborsky, L, Woody, GE, O'Brien, CP, and Druley, KA. 1982. Is treatment for substance abuse effective? *Journal of the American Medical Association* 247:1423–1428.

Metzger, DS, and Platt, JJ. 1988. Solving vocational problems. In *Proceedings of the Dutch-American Conference on the Effectiveness of Drug Abuse Treatment.*

Payte, JT, and Khuri, ET. 1993. Principles of methadone dose determination. In: Center for Substance Abuse Treatment (1992) *State Methadone Treatment Guidelines. Treatment Improvement Protocol (TIP)* Series 1. DHHS Publication No. (SMA) 93-1991. Rockville, Md.:DHHS.

Platt, JJ, and Metzger, DS. 1982. The role of employment in the rehabilitation of heroin addicts. In *Progress in the Development of Cost Effective Treatments.* NIDA Research Monograph 58, Pp. 111–125.

Pond, SM, Kreek, MJ, Tong, TG, Raghunath, J, and Benowitz, NL. 1985. Altered methadone pharmacokinetics in methadone-maintained pregnant women. *Journal of Pharmacology and Experimental Therapeutics* 233:1–6.

Portnoy, RK, and Payne, R. 1992. Acute and chronic pain. In: Lowinson, Ruiz, Millman, and Langrod, (eds.), *Substance Abuse: A Comprehensive Textbook.* 2nd ed. Baltimore: Williams & Wilkins. Pp. 691–721.

Resnik, R. 1983. Methadone detoxification from illicit opiates and methadone maintenance. In: J.R. Cooper, F. Altman, B.S. Brown, et al. (ed.), *Research on the Treamtment of Narcotic Addiction: State of the Art.* Publication No. 9ADM) 83-1281. Rockville, Md.:NIDA, DHHS.

Rounsaville, BJ, Weissman, MM, and Wilber, CH. 1982. The heterogeneity of psychiatric diagnosis in treated opiate addicts. *Archives of General Psychiatry* 39:161–166.

Sells, SB, Demaree, RG, and Hornick, CW. 1979. *Comparative Effectiveness of Drug Abuse Treatment Modalities.* NIDA Service Research Administrative Report. Washington D.C.

Senft, RA. 1991. Kaiser Permanente, Center for Health Research, Experience with clonidine-naltrexone for rapid opiate detoxification. *Journal of Substance Abuse Treatment* 8(4):257–259.

Stanton, MD. 1979. The client as a family member. In B.S. Brown (ed.) *Addicts and Aftercare* New York: Sage.

Stanton, MD, Todd, T, et al. 1992. *The Family Therapy of Drug Abuse and Addiction.* New York: Guilford Press.

Stimmel, B, Goldberg, J, Reisman, A, Murphy, R, and Teets, K. 1982-1983. Fetal outcome in narcotic dependent women: The importance of the type of maternal narcotic used. *American Journal of Drug and Alcohol Abuse* 9(4):383–395.

Woody, GE, McLellan, AT, Luborsky, and L, O'Brien, CP. 1987. Psychotherapy for opiate dependence: A 12-month follow-up. *American Journal of Psychiatry* 145:109–114.

Woody, GE, McLellan AT, Luborsky, L, et al. 1984. Severity of psychiatric symptoms as a predictor of benefits from psychotherapy: The Veterans Administration-Penn Study. *American Journal of Psychiatry* 141(10):1172–1177.

Woody, GE, Luborsky, L, McLellan, AT, et al. 1983. Psychotherapy for opiate addicts: Does it help? *Archives of General Psychiatry* 40:639–345.

Yancovitz, SR, Des Jarlais DC, Peyser, NP, Drew, et al. 1991. *American Journal of Public Health* 81(9):1185–1191.

Zweben, JE, and Payte, JT. 1990. Methadone maintenance in the treatment of opioid dependence: A current perspective. *Western Journal of Medicine* 152(5):588–599.

8

Implementing Standards—and Beyond

The preceding chapter considered the question of how the narcotic addiction treatment standards the Secretary of HHS is obligated to issue, as currently implemented solely by regulations, affect the provision of treatment services, and how these regulations might be changed to encourage optimal clinical practice.

Two additional general issues are dealt with in this chapter. The first deals with the implementation of standards by means that go beyond exclusive reliance on regulations. As noted earlier in the report, regulations have been the exclusive means by which standards have been implemented historically. They need not be the only means. The major approaches identified by the IOM committee for implementing standards are (1) some combination of regulations, clinical practice guidelines, and a formal quality assurance system, or (2) reliance on the existing norms of clinical practice without more regulations.

Reliance on the existing norms of clinical practice is conceptually attractive, as it embodies the proposition that methadone should be treated just like any other medication. Historical experience with methadone, however, cautions that some clinicians can be expected to exploit such a situation for personal gain, and others may act out of ignorance in ways that lead to adverse patient outcomes. Thus, the committee considered and rejected the approach of relying on existing norms.

It is the committee's view that regulations need to be supplemented by some combination of practice guidelines and quality assurance. But improving on the regulations need not wait on the development of infrastructure for guidelines and quality assurance system, nor can the regulations be abandoned entirely.

What follows is intended to provide background for the eventual integration of the three approaches—regulations, guidelines, and quality assurance systems. If standards are to be implemented through a combination of means, what are the appropriate relationships among these means? In the first half of this chapter, we consider the role of regulations and their enforcement, and the concurrent use of clinical practice guidelines and formal quality assurance systems, and conclude by considering steps that can be taken now to achieve the desired balance among them.

The second general topic addresses the need for federal government leadership regarding methadone treatment, especially with respect to research, federal-state relations, treatment financing, and policy guidance. These topics are taken up in the second half of the chapter.

REGULATIONS AND THEIR ENFORCEMENT

A criticism of the methadone regulations has been that they are "process-oriented" and not outcome- or performance-oriented. In 1982, Dole and his colleagues criticized the extensive paperwork required of methadone maintenance treatment programs by federal and state regulatory authorities (Dole et al., 1982). These requirements, they wrote, had resulted in every therapeutic decision being controlled either from Washington or Albany, but had not ensured good quality services and had failed to prevent the flow of methadone to the illicit market. A "more rational approach," they argued, would involve trying "to improve the performance of the clinics" in drug abuse treatment, including "the critical areas" of health, housing, employment, and behavioral problems. They saw no uncertainty about the primary objective of eliminating drug abuse and socially rehabilitating patients, and "no fundamental problem" in measuring achievement of these objectives. They described briefly a performance rating system that they hoped might be adopted and "used constructively" by regulatory agencies.

In 1990, the U.S. General Accounting Office (GAO) issued a report, based on a sample of 24 treatment programs, which found great variation in the "policies, goals, and practices" of methadone maintenance treatment programs. The heart of the GAO criticism was the following: "There are no federal treatment effectiveness standards for treatment programs. Instead, federal regulations are process oriented in that they establish administrative requirements for programs. Even with regard to these requirements, federal oversight of methadone maintenance treatment programs has been very limited since 1982" (GAO, 1990.)

Dole reiterated his criticism in slightly modified terms in 1992. "Guidelines" for clinicians were now viewed favorably, while "process" regulations were still regarded as pernicious in intent and effect. He argued that "a closer linkage of [patient] outcome to [medical] procedure" would be beneficial. Dole found a problem, however, in "the detached attitude of the medical profession," manifest in the absence of medical school teaching about addiction and the contemptuous attitude of senior faculty toward the treatment of addicts. He believed that this attitude was "not likely to persist in the mainstream of medicine beyond this generation," and that a "concerned medical profession" would exert leadership in "setting standards for optimal therapy" as a counterweight to the regulatory bureaucracy.

The critique of the regulations from these various sources thus includes a number of disparate concerns—undue administrative burden, infringement on clinical authority, and the absence of (or adverse) effect upon patient outcomes, program performance, and the quality of services provided. Some criticisms are inconsistent: for example, although the GAO adopted Dole's "process oriented" criticism that the regulations provided no standards of effectiveness, it saw the absence of federal oversight as a problem that implied a federal solution, a decidedly different view from that of Dole.

The IOM committee is sympathetic to the critique of the methadone regulations. It regards the current regulations as unreasonably extensive and intrusive, and finds no compelling *medical* reason for regulating the therapeutic use of methadone differently from any other Schedule II controlled substance. These substances include (see 21 CFR 1308.12) opiates (such as fentanyl, hydrocodone, hydromorphone, meperidine, morphine, and oxycodone), cocaine, stimulants (such as amphetamines and methamphetamines), short-acting central nervous system depressants (such as amobarbital, pentobarbital, phencyclidine, and secobarbital), and hallucinogenic derivatives of marijuana (such as dronabinol and nabicone).

The committee recognizes, however, that historically the regulations were adopted to achieve several competing objectives simultaneously—to make effective treatment available, to minimize the illicit diversion of methadone, and (implicitly) to shield treatment programs from direct public opposition.

In general, regulations establish minimum performance requirements for regulated parties, proscribe certain behaviors, and provide for sanctions when proscribed behaviors occur. They may also exhort regulated parties to nonenforceable good behavior that reflects important community values. However, they also impose a burden they require paperwork; they subject the affected parties to inspections; and they may freeze institutions in place and inhibit innovation.

Thus, the committee is both critical of the methadone regulations in many respects regulations and cognizant that they provide a number of positive benefits. The regulations support methadone treatment, encourage comprehensive care, and provide guidance to state authorities, hospitals, and medical practitioners. Although some believe that these goals can be accomplished by clinical practice guidelines, the committee believes that guidelines alone are not enough to assure that patients are cared for in a safe and thoughtful manner. Methadone treatment is subject to weak scrutiny by patients, who may lack the ability or motive to make rigorous judgments about the treatments, and by payers, who often lack effective means of oversight. Moreover, public support, as noted in chapter 1, is often problematic. **The committee concludes, therefore, that a need exists to maintain certain enforceable requirements in order to deter substandard or unethical practices.**

Generalizing from the specific recommendations made in the discussion of optimal treatment, (see chapter 7) the committee developed the following general principles regarding what regulations should and should not do. These are:

1. Regulations should require that methadone programs approved to treat opiate addiction make comprehensive care available to all opiate-addicted patients entering methadone treatment, either on-site or by referral. The range of services available to patients entering treatment should be specified, especially to those who present with a wide range of medical and psychosocial needs. Optimal care requires attention to the needs of specific patients and to ensuring that those with multiple treatment needs receive the appropriate services, including rehabilitative services. Therefore, *offering methadone with only minimal counseling services on admission is inappropriate for most patients.* Federal regulations should require that licensed programs have the resources on-site or readily available through documented, working, and demonstrated contractual agreement with other agencies to provide for a full range of services for patients accessing treatment.

2. Regulations should emphasize the need for the ongoing clinical assessment of patients throughout the treatment process, rather than arbitrarily specifying periods of treatment time, with respect to the intensity, level, and types of services needed.

3. Regulations should provide clear instructions to programs regarding the procedures for the involuntary administrative withdrawal of medication, termination of treatment, or discharge of patients, whether for disciplinary or other nontherapeutic reasons, such as threatening behavior, drug dealing, and failure to pay fees or follow program rules. These procedures should provide rights of due process to ensure safe and humane treatment of individuals.

4. Regulations should not arbitrarily restrict physician and clinical practice by dictating the length of treatment, establishing rules without scientific or clinical justification, or limiting maximum methadone take-home doses for the sole purpose of controlling methadone diversion without weighing the benefits to the patient against the risks of diversion.

5. Regulations *should not* promote withdrawal from methadone maintenance treatment without regard to the probability that the patient will return to opiate addiction.

6. Regulations *should* prohibit any practice of basing medication dose level on patient participation in or compliance with the treatment program.

In short, the committee does not recommend that the regulations be abandoned. It does recommend that they be reduced in scope and be supplemented clinical practice guidelines and, potentially, by formal quality assurance systems that shift responsibility for treatment decisions from regulators to clinicians. Implementation of this recommendation will also require additional resources, a matter discussed below.

We cannot leave this discussion of regulations, however, without addressing the issues of enforcement. Throughout the study the committee heard complaints, both from its own members and from others, about how the methadone regulations are enforced. Although the report devotes relatively little space to enforcement, this limited coverage should not be understood as a dismissal of its importance. In the committee's judgment, the following points pertaining to enforcement need to be made:

First, DEA should focus its attention on standards for the physical security and recordkeeping associated with the safe handling, storage, and dispensing of opiate medications (including methadone and LAAM), but should have no role controlling or limiting medical practice.

Second, enforcement does entail inspection. And in the multitier methadone treatment regulatory regime, which involves at least two federal agencies, state authorities, and sometimes county and municipal authorities, inspections are time-consuming, costly, redundant, and overlapping.

The committee recommends that the FDA, with SAMHSA and NIDA, conduct an extensive review of methadone enforcement policies, procedures, and practices by all health agencies of government—federal, state, and local—for the purpose of designing a single inspection format, having multiple elements, that would (1) provide the basis for consolidated, comprehensive inspections conducted by one agency (under a delegation of federal authority, if necessary), which serves all agencies and (2) improve the efficiency of the provision of methadone services by reducing the number of inspections and consolidating their purposes.

Third, a need exists to improve the quality of inspections, especially the competence of inspectors with respect to the nature and purpose of methadone treatment programs.

To that end, the committee recommends that the relevant HHS federal regulatory agencies develop an annual training program for inspectors, whether from FDA, DEA, state agencies, or local units of government; that such a training program review all aspects of methadone treatment so that inspections can be more focused and better informed; and that this training program be designed to support the above recommendation of a consolidated review by one agency acting on behalf of all.

Finally, the committee believes that is necessary for an effective enforcement effort to weed out programs that do not meet established standards. The committee does not subscribe to the proposition that any program is better than none. An effective compliance program should close or bring into compliance bad programs. The public expects and deserves as much.

CLINICAL PRACTICE GUIDELINES

The historical reliance on regulations to implement narcotic addiction treatment standards has meant that alternatives have received little conceptual attention. In this section and the next, we consider clinical practice guidelines and formal quality assurance systems as ways to complement reduced-scope regulations and shift responsibility for the provision of treatment services from regulators to clinicians.

Clinical practice guidelines (or "practice parameters," as the American Medical Association calls them) have assumed increasing prominence in health policy since 1989. In that year, the Agency for Health Care Policy and Research (AHCPR) was created with an explicit legislative mandate to develop such guidelines in collaboration with the medical community.

Soon after its creation, AHCPR asked the IOM to advise it on its new guidelines responsibilities. The resulting 1990 IOM report (Field and Lohr, 1990) focused on definitions of terms, attributes of good guidelines, and certain aspects of planning and implementation. A 1992 IOM report (Field and Lohr, 1992) dealt more broadly with the development, implementation, evaluation, and revision of guidelines. The definition of guidelines in the 1990 IOM (Field and Lohr, 1990) report was: "Practice guidelines are systematically developed statements to assist practitioner and patient decisions about appropriate health care for specific clinical circumstances." In addition, the eight attributes of good practice guidelines that this committee identified were validity, reliability and reproducibility, clinical applicability, clinical flexibility, clarity, multidisciplinary process, scheduled review, and documentation.

The AHCPR has issued a number of such guidelines since 1991, including two recent ones dealing with depression in primary care (Depression Guidelines Panel, 1993) and pain management of cancer (Jacox et al., 1994). Medical societies have also taken up guidelines development. For example, the American Academy of Child and Adolescent Psychiatry (AACAP) has issued "practice parameters" for assessing and treating attention-deficit hyperactivity disorder (AACAP, 1991). The American Psychiatric Association (APA), to take another example, issued a "Practice Guideline for Major Depressive Disorder in Adults" (APA, 1993). Similar efforts are under way in many fields of medicine and can be expected to increase in years ahead.

Guidelines are also making their appearance in the substance abuse area. The first instance, as noted in chapter 5, may have been when the 1989 joint FDA-NIDA revision of the methadone regulations removed the language that was discretionary and incorporated it in a guidance document (FDA-NIDA, 1989). Although this document was intended "to provide recommendations" for medical and other services beyond those required by the regulations, it provided no review of or references to the scientific literature.[1] It appeared, as noted above, just as the broader guidelines development was getting under way. The document does not provide a model for guidelines development today, but is notable for being an early indication of movement in this direction.

Although the FDA issues general guidelines for clinical research in many classes of medications, these are not clinical practice guidelines. They state "the formal position of FDA" on a matter and "establish principles or practices of general applicability . . . that are not legal requirements but are acceptable to FDA for a subject matter which falls within the laws administered by the Commissioner" (21 CFR 10.90 (1991)). They bind FDA, if the sponsor of a therapeutic product wishes and agrees, for example, to the design of a Phase III clinical trial or to the endpoints of such a trial in advance of its conduct. FDA guidelines are concerned with the premarket evaluation of therapeutic products and have no binding force on the clinical use of approved products. They provide no model for methadone treatment.

The most promising guidelines-related development in the substance abuse area is the work of the Center for Substance Abuse Treatment (CSAT) of SAMHSA and its Treatment Improvement Protocol (TIP) series. TIPs are described by SAMHSA as "state-of-the-art guidelines for the treatment of alcohol and other drug abuse," which seek to ground substance abuse treatment practice in expert consensus and the scientific literature. (At this time, the

---

[1] The FDA and NIDA made clear that the guidance document did not represent their formal legal opinion," nor was it meant to preclude the states from further regulating the practice of medicine in the treatment of narcotic drug addicts."

CSAT TIP process may emphasize consensus somewhat more than the AHCPR science-oriented guidelines.)

The development of a TIP begins with the identification by agency staff of an alcohol or other drug abuse problem that deserves consideration by experts. A topic, once identified, is reviewed by a federal government resource panel, which frames the questions for review by a second group of nonfederal experts. This second group, called a consensus panel, does the work of reviewing the literature, defining protocols, and making recommendations. Finally, a review group is asked to comment on the work of the second group. The result is a TIP, which is then widely disseminated to the substance abuse treatment community.

In late 1992, CSAT released *State Methadone Treatment Guidelines*, which became the first TIP when republished (CSAT, 1993e). This document provides useful information and recommendations to clinicians, program administrators, state agencies, and federal officials. It takes the federal regulations of methadone as given, and does not recommend the substitution of guidelines for regulations. Currently, a second TIP is under development that addresses the matching of treatment to the type and intensity of services needed. Other TIPs have been prepared dealing with pregnant substance-using women (CSAT, 1993c), treatment of drug-exposed infants (CSAT, 1993b), screening for infectious diseases among substance abusers (CSAT, 1993a) and treating alcohol- and other drug-abusing adolescents (CSAT, 1993a).

The committee regards the TIPs protocols as moving in the general direction of clinical practice guidelines as defined by AHCPR. In general, the TIP process may have reached a point where an overall review of the underlying philosophy and strategy is warranted. If such a review is undertaken, the following issues general issues identified by the 1992 IOM guidelines report (Field and Lohr, 1992) should be considered: the objectives of guidelines, the intended users and their needs, the scope of a guideline, the strength of the scientific and clinical evidence for a guideline, the credibility of the guideline development process (including the acquisition of expert judgment and the reconciliation of differences), the relation of the guidelines to the desired health outcomes, the adaption of national guidelines to local conditions, and the means for evaluating the impact of guidelines.

The committee considered guidelines as an alternative to regulations. However, since the general development of clinical practice guidelines is in its early stages, which is also true for substance abuse and methadone maintenance treatment, a good deal more work must go forward before guidelines can be regarded as an actual alternative to existing regulations.

FORMAL QUALITY ASSURANCE SYSTEMS

Formal quality assurance (QA) systems, either governmental or private, are another way to complement reduced-scope regulations and shift responsibility for the provision of treatment services from regulators to clinicians. The evaluation of quality of care in medicine has relied on the conceptual framework posited nearly 30 years ago by Donabedian, (Donabedian A. Evaluating the quality of Medical Care. *Milbank Memorial Fund Quarterly* 44:166-203, July (Part 2) 1966) in which he identified structural, process, and outcome measures of quality. Although several decades ago attention was focused on structural (or input) measures, the emphasis in recent years has been on patient outcomes and the related processes of care. Assessing quality requires not only measures of outcomes and processes of care, but a way to relate the two, a nontrivial analytical task.

In the substance abuse area, formal QA systems are less well developed than are practice guidelines. The basic issues that need to be considered in the design of a formal QA system include the outcome measures to be used to assess treatment effectiveness; the availability of instruments for measuring outcomes and for adjusting for severity of addiction and illness; the data systems needed to aggregate clinic level data for national and regional evaluative purposes; the relation of data systems to the financing of care; the incentives of providers to submit accurate data to the system; and systematic ways to validate the data. In addition, traditional QA systems have focused on fixed standards of treatment, whereas continuous quality improvement (CQI) is conceptually antithetical to fixed standards and emphasizes continuing improvement in performance. CQI attempts both to reduce the variation around the level of average performance and, at the same time, to improve average performance.

Furthermore, most QA systems are tied in important ways to reimbursement. In the case of Medicare, the incentives for hospitals to participate in QA systems relate to the desire to be paid[2]. Similar reimbursement-related QA systems are now emerging in relation to managed care organizations. In substance abuse treatment, which is financed through federal block grant funds, Medicaid, state, county, and municipal funds, private insurance, and patient's out-of-pocket funds, no single revenue stream provides a strong enough incentive at this time to generate the data required of a formal QA system. This deficiency could possibly change under health care reform if substance abuse treatment is included in the basic benefit package.

---

[2]See Lohr (1990) for a review of the pertinent literature and a discussion of operational systems, such as the Medicare Peer Review Organizations and the Joint Commission on the Accreditation of Healthcare Organization.

An important current effort, sponsored by NIDA, is the Methadone Treatment Quality Assurance System, a research effort now in Phase II of a three-phase study designed to assess the feasibility of a performance-based reporting and feedback system for methadone treatment programs. This effort offers the prospect of laying the foundation for a formal QA system in the future. It is some distance from completion, however, and when complete will have addressed only the research and not the infrastructure questions enumerated above.

WHAT CAN BE DONE NOW?

Steps can be taken now to augment regulations and set the stage for practice guidelines or quality assurance systems. The effectiveness of individual treatment programs can be evaluated by both "process" and "outcomes."

Process Evaluation

Process evaluation requires that quality be assessed by measures of the appropriate patient treatment procedures. The merit of such procedures can be defined independently of the outcomes of care. For example, we suggested in the preceding chapter treatment that patients receiving methadone maintenance treatment should be (1) evaluated comprehensively for their medical, drug and alcohol, psychosocial, criminal, and employment problems; (2) offered on-site (or nearby) medical screening for diseases such as AIDS, other sexually transmitted diseases, tuberculosis, and hepatitis; (3) given on-site counseling by competent and appropriate trained and supervised professionals; and (4) provided on-site (or referrals to) professional medical, mental health, and other social services.

These four processes could form the basis for QA "process criteria" standardized for clinical or administrative use, with time parameters specified for when these procedures should be measured, both initially and on a recurring basis. These QA "process criteria" could be used by a clinic as part of its own internal management practices, but also by independent evaluators as part of annual licensing or other approval review.

Outcome Evaluation

The committee does not recommend outcome-oriented regulations because it does not believe that regulations, with all their rigidities, should be the vehicle for outcome assessment. Nor does it believe that the determinants of methadone treatment outcomes are that well understood. The committee does believe it important to indicate, however briefly, how outcome evaluation might be improved.

The use of process criteria, as indicated in the preceding section, would help standardize the assessment of therapeutic procedures by indicating whether they were done "correctly" or not. But their use does not indicate the effectiveness of the procedures, which must be defined in relation to the public health objectives for methadone maintenance treatment as well as in relation to the well-being of the individuals being treated. These objectives are the elimination of illicit opiate use and reduction of illicit nonopiate drug use; the general increase in positive social behaviors and employment; and the reduction of AIDS-transmission behaviors, crime, social violence, and the disproportionate use of medical and social services.

These goals go beyond simply reducing or even eliminating excessive opiate use. We believe that they reflect public expectations for methadone maintenance treatment and that their achievement can and should be measured in any outcome evaluation. These goals do not imply that every treatment program can be expected to accomplish the full range of these objectives solely with the services it offers, most of which are designed to address some of these expectations but not all of them. Achieving the full range of expectations will require integration and coordination with treatment services that may be provided by other agencies.

Evaluating the effectiveness of a methadone maintenance program, depending on its size, can be done by assessing all patients or by taking a sample of randomly selected patients. In either case, patients are followed from admission to some time later. Given the severity of the problems presented by most patients in methadone treatment and the need for a sustained period of treatment as a prerequisite for "rehabilitative" change, it is important to consider the timing of outcome assessments.

It is inappropriate to consider follow-up evaluation earlier than three months after admission. It is appropriate, however, to measure patient status during the time that the patient is receiving methadone treatment. *Specific time periods should be dealt with in practice guidelines, not regulations.* With respect to such time periods, we believe that an opiate-addicted patient maintained on methadone can be considered a limited "success" at three-, six-, and twelve-month intervals if his or her problems have not required hospitalization and there have been no increases in the severity of his or her medical, criminal justice, economic, family, environment, and substance abuse problems that would encourage relapse.

It is necessary to measure both outcome at a given time and improvement over time, and to distinguish between the two. Outcome as a status measure taken at a single point in time—for example, whether a patient is employed, is using 10 bags of heroin a day, out of treatment—can provide a clear picture of the functional status of a patient at a given time. In contrast, improvement over time requires at least two measurements, typically at admission and some later time during or after treatment. For example, a patient may be found to be working twice as many days as he or she was at admission (or at the earlier measurement time), to be using half as many bags of heroin, and to have been hospitalized on average three days per year less than in the year before treatment. Repeated measures indicate whether the patient has changed in a positive social way during treatment. Both types of information—status at a given time and improvement over time—are important in assessing treatment effectiveness and should be considered together.

Objective measurement for outcomes can be taken in the following ways:

1. Medical/psychiatric—could include laboratory analyses, physical examination results, or at least a record of hospitalizations
2. Alcohol/drug use—repeated, random evaluations with breathalyzer and urinalysis, or at the least a record of hospitalizations for substance abuse disorders
3. Employment—verification via pay stubs or other independent information
4. Crime—arrest records, probation/parole violations

Many evaluations of methadone maintenance focus on patient retention or length of time in treatment. A logical case can be made that treatment retention is a good proxy measure of the ability of a program to engage a patient in rehabilitation and to convince him or her of the need to pursue the specified course of change. At best, however, retention is an indirect measure of the effect of treatment. Other factors, such as court, family, or employer pressure, might be as responsible for treatment retention as the direct efforts of the treatment program itself.

We do not argue against the use of retention as one informative measure of treatment efficacy, only that it should not substitute for direct and valid measures of reduction in opiate and nonopiate drug use and improvement in positive social function. At the same time, retention in treatment is often associated with patient rehabilitation. Thus, most patients improve if they remain in methadone maintenance treatment for one or more years, during which time they are encouraged, supported, and monitored in their rehabilitation.

FEDERAL GOVERNMENT LEADERSHIP

The second broad question raised in this chapter—what is needed beyond standards?—brings us to the topic of federal government leadership. This topic involves the issues of research, federal-state relations, the financing of substance abuse treatment, especially as it pertains to the use of methadone, and the need for policy guidance on substance abuse treatment within the Department of Health and Human Services.

Research Issues

Although the methadone regulations affect primarily the provision of treatment services, they also affect the conduct of research. Since that another IOM committee was examining the NIDA Medications Development Program concurrent with this study, this committee devoted relatively limited attention to research questions.

There are two issues, however, on which the committee wishes to comment. The first, which was addressed by the IOM committee that reported on the NIDA Medications Development Program, (see IOM, 1994), involves the constraints imposed by the methadone regulations on the conduct of clinical research. The second pertains to the requirement contained in the ADAMHA Reorganization Act of 1992 that 15 percent of the NIDA research budget be spent on health services research.

Clinical Research

Research involving the use of a new drug in human subjects, or a new application of a previously approved drug, is conducted under the Investigational New Drug (IND) regulations of FDA. If the drug in question is a controlled substance, such as methadone, LAAM, or any other opiate agonist, or if a controlled substance is used in the comparison treatment in a clinical trial in which the drug of interest is not a controlled substance, such research must still comply with the three-tiered regulation by FDA and the DEA described in detail in chapter 5.

DEA regulations under the Controlled Substances Act require registration, specific kinds of recordkeeping, and periodic reporting. DEA also requires that protocols for research involving schedule I controlled substances not conducted under an IND (preclinical studies) be approved by it (see IOM, 1994, pp. 74–76, for a detailed discussion).

The effect of DEA regulation, as noted by the report of the IOM committee on NIDA medications development (IOM, 1994), is to create "a clinical research environment for scheduled drugs that is extraordinarily bureaucratic from the procedural point of view and unnecessarily difficult, given the low public health risk associated with diversion" in research conducted under the IND regulations of FDA.

The present committee concurs in the basic judgment of medications development committee that this DEA regulation of clinical research is an unnecessary impediment to the conduct of such research. Since clinical research is essential to the development of new scientific and clinical information, from which answers to problems of drug addiction can be expected to emerge, we regard these regulations as contrary to the public interest.

The IOM committee on NIDA medications development made the following recommendation (IOM, 1994):

The committee recommends that action be taken to remove the adverse effects of DEA requirements, under the Controlled Substances Act (CSA), on clinical research involving controlled substances, by holders of active FDA INDs, either by amending the CSA to exempt such investigations from applicable DEA regulations or by the alternative administrative and regulatory measures:

- The development of a Memorandum of Understanding between FDA and DEA governing the matter of dual authority over clinical research to provide exemption from DEA reporting requirements.
- DEA revision of 21 CFR 1301.22 and parallel regulations to provide that protocols, drug security, recordkeeping, production controls, reporting, and other requirements would be governed by the FDA regulations and monitored by FDA. This would require parallel changes in FDA's IND regulations.

This committee endorses the above recommendation.

Health Services Research

The ADAMHA Reorganization Act of 1992 required that 15 percent of the research funds of the National Institutes of Mental Health, National Institute of Alcoholism and Alcohol Abuse, and National Institute of Drug Abuse be spent in health services research. In the case of NIDA, compliance with this requirement will undoubtedly involve research on the delivery of substance abuse treatment services, some of which may involve methadone or LAAM or other controlled substances.

In such investigations, it is unlikely that the medication itself will be the object of research. Rather, the issue will be how best to deliver treatment using such a medication. Such research may involve comparing the treatment setting, inpatient or outpatient, and, if the latter, whether a clinic or a physician's office is the most appropriate location for treatment. It may also involve the evaluation or assessment of the criteria for rewarding successful treatment by the granting of take-home privileges in the case of methadone, or it may also involve other health services research issues. For example, a project might examine treatment effectiveness and cost of care by providing pharmacy-based dispensing for methadone patients who have three years of perfect compliance (no opiate-positive urines) and lead stable lives.

It is necessary that such health services research be permitted to experiment with various institutional arrangements and that it not be subjected a priori to regulations that force it into a pattern prescribed by the methadone regulations. That is to say, if drug delivery in such research must comply with existing methadone regulations, we will never learn whether there are safer and more effective ways to treat addiction using alternative means of drug delivery, or whether these alternative means affect the potential for drug diversion and abuse.

The committee recommends that NIDA, in conjunction with SAMHSA and FDA, develop a general policy to guide health services research involving controlled substances such as methadone and LAAM, and negotiate a memorandum of understanding with the DEA to govern such research.

Federal-State Relations

The regulation, financing, and provision of treatment services for substance abuse, usually including drug and alcohol abuse, involves shared responsibilities between the federal government and the states. For example, the federal methadone regulations, including those of both FDA and DEA, rely on active participation by the states for the approval of treatment program applications, the revocation of program registrations, and certain other decisions.

In partial response to these federal requirements, a substantial state administrative, regulatory, and financing apparatus has been established in the two decades since methadone was first approved for use in treatment of opiate addiction. In addition to substance abuse responsibilities, the states also exercise their traditional functions of licensure of professional personnel engaged in the provision of clinical services.

Although the federal regulations establish a common framework regarding methadone treatment services, great variation is found among the states regarding methadone treatment services. Variations in state policies and procedures appears to be unrelated to state variation in prevalence of opiate addiction and in the characteristics of the treated patient population described in chapter 3.

The report summarizes state rules in five jurisdictions—New York, California, Massachusetts, Illinois, and Florida—in Chapter 6, but does not go beyond this limited analysis. As noted in Chapter 1, however, a comprehensive description does not exist of the authorities and agencies of the states that govern medications that may be used for treatment of opiate addiction. Based on these five case studies, the knowledge of committee members, and anecdotal information acquired during the study, there appear to be three broad groups into which the several states fall. First, some states have adopted policies that are essentially consistent with the federal regulations. Second, another group of states regulate the provision of methadone treatment services more strictly than does the federal government, or in ways that are inconsistent with federal regulations as presently written. Third, some states provide no treatment services. The issues of federal–state relations vary for each grouping.

In the states whose regulations and policies are the same as those of the federal government, federal regulations provide a framework or a policy baseline regarding treatment at the state government level. State decisions about financing and regulating treatment are consistent with the federal regulations. These states are apt to be receptive to technical assistance, including that provided by clinical practice guidelines. They are likely to take a strong interest in the availability and constructive use of federal funds for treatment programs. They are candidates for a contractual delegation of the compliance and investigation function from the federal government.

Other states impose more severe restrictions on methadone treatment services than do the federal regulations. Their regulations may discourage or restrict services, for example, by limiting the length of time a patient can receive methadone treatment, by limiting the maximum dose of methadone that may be prescribed, by prohibiting take-home medication, or by capitating reimbursement or restricting it to short-term treatment having "abstinence" as a primary goal. For the same reasons cited with respect to the federal methadone regulations, these state policies limit access to treatment and impair its quality.

States that provide no treatment services represent a different situation. No language in the federal regulations requires that individual states provide methadone services for its opiate-addicted patients. Nine states have no methadone treatment services.

Both philosophical and financial factors lie behind state policies to limit or deny access to methadone treatment services. Some state agencies (as well as some managed care companies) not only insist that a drug-free approach, i.e., abstinence, is preferable, but that it is the only efficacious treatment approach despite the absence of supporting data. In these cases, an understandable preference for a drug-free outcome of treatment has hardened into an ideological premise that ignores clinical evidence about the effectiveness of methadone treatment and the likelihood of relapse to opiate use when patients are withdrawn from such treatment.

This study focused on federal methadone regulations, but the experience with LAAM, which was approved by the FDA in 1993 for use in the treatment of narcotic addiction, highlights the extensive web of the state regulatory apparatus for substance abuse prevention, treatment, financing, and control. The requirements for approval of the use of this medication began at the federal level but now extend to a labyrinth of state agency requirements, which often differ from state to state, involve multiple agencies, and are subject to numerous local political interests. Massachusetts, for example, has to adopt a state regulation that permits the use of LAAM, an FDA-approved medication, for the treatment of opiate addiction.

In a memorandum of November 4, 1993, addressed to Dr. Frank Vocci of the NIDA Medications Development Program, among others, H. Alex Bradford, chief executive officer of the BioDevelopment Corporation, the commercial sponsor of LAAM, outlined the complexity of the state approval process. He identified "five general areas" that needed to be addressed before an individual clinic (i.e., treatment program) could purchase LAAM:

1. Existing state treatment regulations, which covered methadone, needed to be modified for LAAM, which in many states requires legislation unless an interim administrative process is employed.

2. The rescheduling of LAAM from a schedule I to schedule II controlled substance under state law is required in many states.

3. The addition of LAAM to the state formulary of medications approved for treating opiate dependence is required.

4. LAAM needed to be included in the list of reimbursable medications for treating opioid dependence.

5. The approval of LAAM's use in the clinic by county and local organizations having responsibility for overseeing the treatment clinics in their jurisdiction is often required.

State regulation of methadone treatment is beyond the scope of this report, but the committee's examination of federal methadone regulations forced it to consider this subject. Although there are too few data to make a detailed assessment of the effect of state regulatory requirements on substance abuse treatment, the committee did arrive at several general conclusions.

First, in fulfilling the standard-setting function of the HHS Secretary, there is a need to maintain a federal system of regulations that proscribe certain activities, such as using medication doses to reward or punish patient's behavior, or failing to provide due process for involuntary administrative termination of treatment. In addition, guidelines should be actively developed to describe good clinical practice in methadone treatment, with state substance abuse authorities in mind as a primary user audience.

Second, the federal government should actively attempt to minimize the administrative burden associated with both federal and state government regulation of methadone treatment. It should seek compatibility of federal and state regulations, and should adopt uniform procedures that allow inspections by one level of government to be satisfactory for other levels. It should, as appropriate, consider the delegation of the inspection and compliance function to the states on a contract basis.

Third, federal regulations should encourage states, through their licensing boards, to assure that medical, nursing, psychological, social work, and pharmacy practitioners have adequate educational training to provide the appropriate care in methadone treatment programs.

Fourth, federal regulations should prohibit states that receive federal funding from developing regulations or contractual requirements that arbitrarily limit services and deny methadone pharmacotherapy to patients who require concurrent treatment for psychiatric illness or other addictions. SAMHSA should be authorized and directed to tie compliance with this requirement to eligibility for block grant funding.

Finally, state regulation of substance abuse treatment is so extensive that the committee recommends that a comprehensive assessment of state substance abuse treatment regulations be undertaken, especially as they pertain to the treatment of opiate addiction, with an eye to developing a model state approach to the financing, treatment, and regulation of services.

Financing of Treatment

The committee was not asked to examine the financing of care, and the data on financing of methadone treatment, discussed in chapter 6, do not permit it to make any authoritative judgments about the adequacy of financing. However, a recent paper by Etheridge et al. (forthcoming) comparing TOPS data for 1979–1981 and DATOS data for 1991–1993 showed a marked decrease in the number and variety of services clients reported receiving. Of four treatment modalities (methadone maintenance, long-term residential, outpatient drug-free, and short-term inpatient), methadone maintenance patients reported the lowest level of drug abuse counseling and services. In addition, the personal experiences of many committee members indicate that resource constraints are substantial in many treatment programs.

Financial barriers to treatment exist for opiate-dependent patients and remain a major barrier for patients awaiting admission to methadone treatment programs. Some states provide no state funding for indigent patients. In others, Medicaid does not reimburse methadone treatment for women with dependent children or patients with disabilities. Others rely on the patient's ability to pay out-of-pocket for services, resulting in high program fees, limited treatment services, and involuntary discharges for those who cannot finance their care. Although there are currently federal block grant monies to improve access to treatment, in the judgment of the committee they do not appear to meet the current treatment demand. These financing limitations create serious barriers to treatment for many patients.

The committee notes two developments that pertain to treatment financing and the underlying concern of this report. First, the fiscal year 1995 budget submission sent to Congress by President Clinton in early 1994 requested increased funding for drug treatment services relative to law enforcement activities. Second, the crime bill passed by Congress in 1994 emphasizes prevention and treatment of substance abuse. It is hoped that increased federal funds will flow to substance abuse treatment services in the near future.

Therefore, the committee recommends that HHS conduct a review of its priorities in substance abuse treatment, including methadone treatment, in a way that integrates changes in regulations and the development of practice guidelines with decisions about treatment financing.

Policy Guidance

The current organization of the Department of HHS for substance abuse prevention, treatment, and research includes the Office of Drug Policy in the Office of the Secretary, the Office of the Assistant Secretary for Health, and, within the Public Health Service, the Food and Drug Administration, the Substance Abuse and Mental Health Services Administration the National

Institute of Drug Abuse, and the National Institute of Alcoholism and Alcohol Abuse.

The HHS agencies concerned with methadone include SAMHSA, NIDA, and FDA. These agencies are coordinated for information exchange purposes by the Interagency Methadone Policy Review Board. Other departments and agencies having both general drug abuse and specific methadone responsibilities include DEA (within the Department of Justice) and the Office of National Drug Control Policy in the Executive Office of the President. These agencies also participate in the discussions of the interagency board.

The current organization of drug abuse policy within the Department of HHS, as revealed in the area of methadone, results in department policy emerging from the independent activities of the pertinent Public Health Service agencies and from coordination between these agencies. The committee concludes that federal policy toward methadone treatment, and in all likelihood broader areas of drug abuse treatment, would benefit from sustained *department-level policy oversight, informed by a clinical perspective,* on all issues relation to regulations, practice guidelines, and treatment financing.

The committee does not believe that such a policy oversight role requires a major organizational change within the Department of HHS. Rather, the committee believes that one official in the Office of the Assistant Secretary for Health should be designated to serve this function for the department. In this respect, the committee reaches a similar conclusion on the need for federal government leadership as did the IOM committee on the NIDA medications development program (see IOM, 1994).

> **The committee recommends that the Secretary of HHS direct the Assistant Secretary for Health to designate one high-level official in the Office of the Assistant Secretary to be responsible for policy oversight and guidance on methadone treatment and on related drug abuse prevention and treatment issues.**

SUMMARY

The committee believes that essential improvements in the regulation of methadone treatment services can be implemented today, and it has chosen to pursue this approach. It finds no reason to delay recommending reasonable reforms until the infrastructure for a "outcomes-oriented" or guidelines based approach is developed. On the other hand, especially given the prospect of health care reform and the possible inclusion of substance abuse in the basic benefit package, we commend the Public Health Service's current efforts to develop such systems in anticipation of their implementation in the near future.

The committee is highly supportive of guidelines and of an outcomes approach and a formal QA system for methadone treatment and believes that these options should be explored aggressively. However, the development of guidelines and the assessment of patient outcomes in medical care is in an early stage and not sufficiently robust to provide an alternative to the current system. These other approaches must complement regulations rather than be advanced as replacements for them.

REFERENCES

American Academy of Child and Adolescent Psychiatry. 1991. AACAP official action: practice parameters for the assessment and treatment of attention-deficit hyperactivity disorder." *Journal of the American Academy of Child and Adolescent Psychiatry* 30(3):i–ii.

American Psychiatric Association. 1993. Practice guideline for major depressive disorder in adults. *American Journal of Psychiatry* 150(4) (Supplement).

Center for Substance Abuse Treatment (CSAT). 1993a. *Guidelines for the Treatment of Alcohol- and Other Drug (AOD)-Abusing Adolescents: The Recommendations of a Consensus Panel.* Treatment Improvement Protocol. Rockville, Md.: U.S. Department of Health and Human Services. Draft.

CSAT. 1993b. *Improving Treatment for Drug-Exposed Infants: The Recommendations of a Consensus Panel.* Treatment Improvement Protocol. Rockville, Md.: U.S. Department of Health and Human Services. Draft.

CSAT. 1993c. *Pregnant Substance-Using Women.* Treatment Improvement Protocol Series 2, Rockville, Md.: U.S. Department of Health and Human Services. (Draft)

CSAT. 1993d. *Screening for Infectious Diseases Among Substance Abusers: The Recommendations of a Consensus Panel.* Treatment Improvement Protocol. Rockville, Md.: U.S. Department of Health and Human Services. Draft

CSAT. 1993e. *State Methadone Treatment Guidelines.* Treatment Improvement Protocol Series 1. Rockville, Md.: U.S. Department of Health and Human Services.

Depression Guideline Panel. 1993. *Depression in Primary Care: Volume 1. Detection and Diagnosis. clinical Practice Guideline No. 5.* AHCPR Publication No. 93-0550. Rockville, Md.: Agency for Health Care Policy and Research, Public Health Service, U.S. Department of Health and Human Services.

Dole, V. 1992. Hazards of process regulations: The example of methadone maintenance. *Journal of the American Medical Association* 267:2234–2235.

Dole, VP, Nyswander, ME, Des Jarlais, D and Joseph, H. 1982. Performance-based rating of methadone maintenance programs. *New England Journal of Medicine* 306:169–172.

Etheridge, RM, Craddock, SG, Dunteman, GH, and Hubbard, RL. Forthcoming. Treatment services in two national studies of community-based drug abuse treatment programs. *Journal of Substance Abuse.*

FDA-NIDA. 1989. Use of Methadone in Maintenance and Detoxification Treatment of Narcotic Addicts. Guidance document issued by the Center for Drug Evaluation and Research of the Food and Drug Administration and the National Institute on Drug Abuse.

Field, MJ, and Lohr, KN, eds. 1990. *Clinical Practice Guidelines: Directions for a New Program.* Washington, D.C.: National Academy Press.

Field, MJ, and Lohr, KN, eds. 1992. *Guidelines for Clinical Practice: From Development to Use.* Washington, D.C: National Academy Press.

General Accounting Office. 1990. *Methadone Maintenance: Some Treatment Programs Are Not Effective; Greater Federal Oversight Needed,* GAO\HRD-90-104, Washington, D.C.: U.S. Government Printing Office.

Institute of Medicine. 1994. *Development of Anti-Addiction Medications: Issues for the Government and Private Sector,* Washington, D.C.: National Academy of Sciences Press.

Jacox, A, Carr, DB, Payne, R, et al. 1994. *Management of Cancer Pain. Clinical Practice Guideline No. 9.* AHCPR Publication No. 94-0592. Rockville, Md.: Agency for Health Care Policy and Research, Public Health Service, U.S. Department of Health and Human Services.

Lohr, KN, ed. 1990. *Medicare: A Strategy for Quality Assurance, Volumes I and II.* Washington, D.C.: National Academy Press.